OPTIMIZE YOUR HEART

A practical guide to lowering your risk of a heart attack or stroke

Andy Beal

Andy Beal/Marketing Pilgrim LLC
9650 Strickland Rd, #103-224
Raleigh, NC 27614
www.andybeal.fitness

Book Layout © 2020 BookDesignTemplates.com
Edited by Lisa Lickel

Optimize Your Heart / Andy Beal. -- 1st ed.
ISBN 9798676594626

For all the doctors, nurses, and caregivers who work tirelessly to help those battling cardiovascular disease.

CONTENTS

Part Three: Exercise Your Cardiac Muscle

Foreword

According to the World Health Organization, the leading cause of death worldwide is heart disease, followed by stroke as a close second. Hence, it can be easily deduced that disease of the arteries of the heart and the brain, as a common denominator, is the primary universal cause of death.

Aside from being a major cause of death, stroke is the leading factor for disability in the United States.

As a stroke physician, I have experienced firsthand how devastating a stroke can be to a person's life, to a family's structure, or even to the community in general.

It is sad enough that this disease leads to sudden death and the loss of loved ones. It is often just as devastating when it takes someone who is fully functional, carrying on their daily activities of being a director at their office, an activist in their community, or even practicing their family member role as a parent or a grandparent, rendering them, in a blink of an eye, disabled, unable to walk, communicate, or even take care of their basic daily needs.

Stroke can transfer a fully functional individual into a fully dependent one overnight, thus ruining a family's makeup and burdening their community with massive financial and social hardships each year.

Heart disease in a very similar way affects communities all over the world albeit on a much larger scale.

Despite all the pharmacological, technical, and medical device advancements we have in the world of cardiac disease and stroke, we continue to be limited in our ability to halt the initial damage caused by them.

While it is extremely rewarding for a doctor to reverse the effects of a stroke or heart attack, save his patient's life, or restore the function of their arm, leg, or their language, we still, as physicians, have a lot of limitations. Sometimes, we feel that we need to move mountains to help our patients.

In the most advanced clinical trials that study stroke victims, using clot-busting medications or cutting-edge devices to target the removal of clots from the brain, only 50% of patients are fortunate enough to return to or close to their baseline. This means that 50% do not! Fifty percent will have lingering symptoms of difficulty finding words, walking, or being independent enough to feed or bathe themselves. A considerable number of these patients won't be fortunate enough to go back home to their families but rather have to stay in nursing homes for continuous professional help.

The old proverb "prevention is better than the cure" can't apply perfectly to anything more than it does to cerebrovascular and heart diseases.

You are what you eat? Yes! Your body is what you eat, furthermore, your arteries are what you eat.

Our arteries are the highways that transmit oxygen and nutrients to our heart muscles and brain neurons. If these arteries become clogged, our tissues, especially those of the heart and brain start suffering, suffocating, and may in time die.

Our arteries' health is reflected by our diet, physical activity, and lifestyle. The better we treat our highways—our arteries—the more "mileage" we can get from them. The healthier they are, the healthier we are.

They say experience is the best teacher, well, the author of this book, Andy Beal, would know a thing or two about that. As a stroke and heart attack survivor, Andy lived through the journey that victims of both of these malicious ailments go through.

He battled disabilities from both simultaneously and managed to emerge victorious, healthful, and eager to do more. He took what he gathered from experience and transferred it to help others. His experience revolves around prevention and eliminating the risks of vascular disease as early as possible to avoid suffering from a heart attack or a stroke. And to live healthier while at it!

I say, why would one go to war to win, when one can avoid the war altogether?

As a health professional, I feel that this book gives the reader a balanced, right-to-the-point summary of the best practices for a healthy heart, a healthy brain, and a healthy life.

As a doctor, I couldn't have said it better myself.

Omar Kass-Hout, MD, MPH

Neuroendovascular Surgery

Medical Director of Stroke and interventional Neurology

UNC REX Hospital

I Hope My Story is Your Inspiration

On April 19, 2018 I did what most normal 44-year-old men do at four o'clock in the morning. I got up to go to the bathroom. What happened next was anything but normal. My entire right side went numb, and I collapsed, barely able to make it to my bed. I woke my wife and told her something was wrong. Something didn't feel right. Little did I know, I was having a mini-stroke.

Having a mini-stroke didn't feel right because I did not expect it to strike at such a young age. Of course, most of my adult life I had been aware of the risks I faced for cardiovascular disease. I had high blood pressure, elevated cholesterol, I was obese, and just one day shy of his 54th birthday, my father died of cardiac arrest. All of those were warning signs, but having a stroke at age 44 never crossed my mind.

What had crossed my mind was the possibility of having a heart attack once I reached my mid-50s. Just eight months before my 4 a.m. wake-up call I decided to get into better shape. I changed my diet, started working out with a personal trainer, and lost 50 pounds. I really believed that I had started to reverse my likelihood of having any acute cardiovascular condition. And yet, I was having a mini-stroke? Surely, that was a misdiagnosis. It wasn't, and my condition was about to get worse. Much, much worse.

Just a few hours later, as is common after a mini-stroke, things escalated. I had a full-blown stroke. Two clots in the carotid artery on the left side of my neck were blocking the flow of blood to half of my brain. The clock was ticking. If the clots were not removed quickly, I could permanently lose all mobility on the right side of my body. Worse case, I would die. Thankfully, hospitals in the Raleigh-Durham region of North Carolina are some of the best in the world. After a quick helicopter transfer, Duke University Hospital neurologists evaluated me with a series of CT scans and MRIs and decided I was a candidate for a new thrombectomy procedure that just recently finished clinical trials and had only been used on two percent of all stroke patients nationwide. The odds were seemingly not in my favor.

As they prepped me for surgery, I watched the frenzy going on around me. I saw the anguish in my wife's eyes but was not sure why. My brain could not comprehend even the simplest of questions asked of me during my evaluation, yet right before I was given the anesthetic that would send me into what could have been my final sleep, a sense of clarity and peace washed over me. I prayed to God that I trusted that my life was in His hands and if my time was up, then I look forward to being in His presence. God had other plans for me.

When I awoke, I felt different. I felt somewhat normal. I could move my right arm and leg. The next few hours involved test after test, evaluation after evaluation. My mobility slowly returned. My speech was more coherent. I wasn't even a full day post-surgery when I started to eat and move around my ICU room unaided. The following day, I walked out of the hospital unassisted. The neurologists were amazed. They called it a "remarkable recovery." It was a miracle.

Still baffled by what caused my stroke, an investigatory MRI and angiogram were conducted on my heart. The results showed that I'd also had a small heart attack and one of my major arteries was 70 percent blocked. A stent opened it back up and they implanted a heart monitor to keep an eye on things for a few more years. A heart attack and a stroke? How on earth had I survived?

To this day, I believe that if not for my decision, just eight months earlier, to improve my heart health, I would not have recovered as fully as I did. I may not even be here. After I passed the 90-day recovery window where the risk is greatest for a second stroke, I decided to double-down on my heart health. I added more strength training, started running, completing two half-marathons, and even hit the mountain bike trails a few times each week.

Not only did I increase my physical activity, I tightened up my diet even further. My friends would come to know me as the Salmon Guy, as it appeared salmon salads were all I would allow on my plate—and post photos to Instagram. I lost an additional 50 pounds in body fat and gained over 15 pounds of additional muscle.

It was then that I realized the new mission laid out before me: to help others improve their heart health.

I became an ambassador for the American Heart Association and American Stroke Association. I wrote dozens of articles. I spoke at medical conferences and fundraisers. I shared heart health tips on social media. I ultimately studied to become a certified personal trainer and weight management specialist so that I could help anyone, at any age, reduce their risk of a heart attack or stroke.

And yet, something was still missing. As a personal trainer, I could only help so many clients each week. I needed a broader, deeper reach. It was time to write a book.

There are hundreds of articles, websites, and books that provide a wealth of information about cardiovascular disease. Even a visit to your primary care physician will be all you need to learn that a bad diet, lack of exercise, or unhealthy habits can contribute to the narrowing of your arteries, higher blood pressure, stroke, heart attack, or cardiac arrest. What's hard to find is a simple, practical guide that sets aside the biology lectures, forgoes unfeasible dietary restrictions, and doesn't insist that you blast every muscle of your body until you are sore, head-to-toe. This is where *Optimize Your Heart* fills the void.

As you read through *Optimize Your Heart*, you will see a book that is laid out in three separate parts, each designed to guide you through your journey to better heart health.

Part One: Cardiac Prehabilitation – Five chapters that are designed to help identify your risk factors, understand why your medical care provider is an important ally, techniques for building healthy habits, and advice for growing your support network.

Part Two: Your Wellness Comes First – If you made just one improvement to your heart health, then focusing on your wellness is a good place to start. You'll learn the foundation of heart-healthy nutrition, why sleep is so important, techniques for reducing stress, and ideas for kicking the bad habits that are sabotaging your cardiovascular system.

Part Three: Exercise Your Cardiac Muscle – Your heart is a muscle that needs exercise. Just about any kind of exercise can be beneficial, but in these chapters, you will be guided to the best physical activity for you, how to set up a training plan you look forward to consistently following, and workout tips that I wish someone had shared with me when I first started.

You are unique. So is your heart. And so, too, is your blueprint for improving your heart health. *Optimize Your Heart* is not a replacement for the advice you receive from your doctor, it's a starting point. Whether you're 34, 44, 54, or 64 years of age, *Optimize Your Heart* is a practical guide to help you reduce your cardiovascular disease risks, eliminate unhealthy habits, improve your nutrition, become more physically active, and optimize your heart health before a stroke or heart attack can strike.

I'm still 100 percent committed to improving my heart health. I am in the best physical shape of my life, sleep well, have more energy, and continually receive glowing reports from my cardiologist and neurologist. Having an optimized heart feels wonderful.

It's a journey without end, but that's a good thing. When you start your journey to optimize your heart, you push life's finish line further and further away. My hope is that *Optimize Your Heart* is exactly what you need to improve your heart health, reduce your risk for cardiovascular disease, prevent a stroke or heart attack, and feel wonderful for the rest of your life.

Part One: Cardiac Prehabilitation

Start Your Healthiest Life Now

It would be easy for me to start the first paragraph of the first chapter by scaring you with all of the studies and research that demonstrate why it's important to optimize your heart health as soon as possible to prevent a heart attack or stroke. Don't worry, I will get to that, but before I do, I would like to start by congratulating you on taking the first step towards optimizing your heart: you've bought this book! Family, friends, websites, and doctors have nagged at you for years about the numerous cardiovascular risks you could face but something—be it a personal epiphany, seeing someone else's battle with heart disease, or perhaps a worrying health scare yourself—has lit a spark inside you that is smoldering so strongly that you are ready to take everything you've been told to do and finally turn it into action!

The Facts of Death

Okay, so I started with the most important section of this chapter: the praise. Now, unfortunately, we need to revisit some cold, morbid facts. Facts that perhaps you already know, perhaps you've never read, or perhaps you have tried to ignore up until today. Cardiovascular disease is the leading cause of mortality in the world, according to the World Health Organization (WHO), accounting for more than 31 percent of all deaths in 2017. That term, cardiovascular disease, covers a myriad of different diseases and conditions, but a 2011 study published by WHO, the World Heart Federation, and the World Stroke Organization reported, of those who die from cardiovascular disease, a staggering 80 percent of men and 75 percent of women die from two types specifically: heart attacks and strokes. That translates to almost 800,000 Americans each year—more than one in every four deaths in the United States.

A sobering thought? Yes, but I am not going to conceal from you an equally important, positive statistic. The Centers for Disease Control and Prevention (CDC) estimates that up to 90 percent of all cardiovascular disease is preventable. Ninety percent! How encouraging is that stat? I hope your answer is "immensely!"

As you make your way through *Optimize Your Heart*, you will learn about the scientifically proven methods YOU can employ to improve your heart health and reduce your risk of a stroke or heart disease. I recognize how that last sentence can read a little like some kind of fake headline you often see in an ad on a website, a magazine, or YouTube video. Don't be alarmed. There will be no snake oil sold to you when discussing the different ways to improve your heart health. Instead, *Optimize Your Heart* will look at simple, practical, ways to improve your cardiovascular health, including eating healthy, sleeping well, reducing stress, breaking bad habits, and keeping active.

The key is to embrace heart disease prevention instead of waiting for heart disease recovery.

Cardiac Prehabilitation

Is that a typo in the above subheading? You would be forgiven for thinking that. Even Microsoft Word spelling and grammar proofreading has added a wiggly red line to the word prehabilitation because it believes I meant to type rehabilitation. That goes to show just how underutilized prehabilitation is in the world of health and wellness.

The word prehabilitation—just like rehabilitation is often shortened to rehab, so too we will shorten prehabilitation to prehab—is somewhat obscurely used in the medical world to describe efforts to improve patients' health before a surgical procedure to reduce their postoperative recovery time. In the world of cardiovascular disease, you won't hear the phrase "cardiac prehab" but you will certainly hear the phrase "cardiac rehab." I know I did after it was discovered, post-stroke, that I had a 70 percent blockage in the left anterior descending artery of my heart. I was assigned a 12-week program to rehabilitate my heart and try to get me back to the best health possible. Fortunately, I had inadvertently invented my own cardiac prehab by taking control of my health eight months before my stroke and angioplasty. As a result, I was barely into my second week of rehab when the cardiac nurse agreed that I was already back to full health and did not need to complete the program.

The concept of cardiac prehab is the main reason I decided to write *Optimize Your Heart*. My goal is to provide encouragement, guidance, and motivation for you, dear reader, to take preventative action now, before you have a heart attack or stroke. Cardiac prehab means taking action to improve your diet, to remove stress and toxic habits, and to find an exercise plan that is not only practical but enjoyable and sustainable. Yes, these changes can cost a little of your time, money, and attention. However, don't think of them as a cost, but as an investment. Just like retirement savings.

Invest in Your Heart

By the time I was discharged from the hospital, my medical bills were north of $200,000. I know that sounds astronomical, but it could have been so much higher. Had I not invested in my health ahead of my stroke, I would have likely spent weeks—perhaps months or years—in a stroke recovery center. My insurance would have covered the vast majority of my medical bills, but there would have been so many more expenses needed to be paid in order to get me back to some semblance of health.

Now relate that to retirement savings. If you retired with nothing but Social Security to cover your retirement expenses, you might get by for a little while. Then the extra costs add up. Hopefully, you are already wise to the hidden costs of retirement and so have started a 401(k) or IRA and are investing, little by little, each month so that you are preemptively building up your nest egg to not only cover any senior expenses but also live your best life at retirement.

The same should be said about your heart health.

Investing in your heart should start as early as possible. Just like retirement, the earlier you start investing in your heart, the healthier you will be to enjoy time with your precious family, go on those scenic hikes you enjoy, or take that cruise around the world! If you wait until after a heart attack or stroke, before you optimize your heart, then it may be too little too late. The risks associated with a heart attack or stroke can often start earlier than you think, and they may be hiding in plain sight.

Application

Write down all of the reasons that sparked your desire to optimize your heart health. Use that as a reminder as you start your journey.

2

Your Risk Factors Are as Unique as You

I'm guessing you already feel you know your risk factors for cardiovascular disease and are perhaps thinking of skipping this chapter. I can't say I blame you. For years, I thought I knew all of my risk factors for heart disease and stroke, yet I would still brush them off as something to worry about when I neared retirement age. Even though my own father died of a massive heart attack just one day before his 54th birthday, it would be another ten years before I accepted that I needed to investigate, acknowledge, and attempt to mitigate all of the cardiovascular disease risk factors while I still had time on my side. I still believe my awakening came just in time, but I wish I had been even more accepting of my risk factors at an earlier age and more aggressive in reducing them before they became a reality, more than just a risk.

Please don't skip over this chapter. I will keep it succinct and to the point. And, while it would be impractical to explore every single risk factor for a heart attack or stroke, I will attempt to draw your attention to those which the CDC, American Heart Association, and, likely, your doctor agree are the ones you should not ignore.

The Risks You Can't Change

There are some cardiovascular disease risks that you simply cannot control or reduce, but they are still a reality, and, once acknowledged, they will become a motivational force that will always push you towards your goal of optimizing your heart.

Your Gender – Sorry gents, but being born a male means you have a much greater risk for heart disease than females. Different studies show different reasons for this increased risk—the most common being men handle stress a lot worse than women. However, ladies, you are not free and clear. While your risk for a stroke or heart attack may be lower, it is still a real risk that cannot be ignored.

Your Family – Ah, yes. How many times has someone commented you have your mother's eyes? Your father's sporting attributes? Your grandmother's compassion? Or, your great-grandfather's leadership skills? You love to hear those compliments. Yet, you can also inherit many things from previous generations that can increase your risk of cardiovascular disease. Medical conditions such as high blood pressure (when the force of the blood pushing against the walls of your blood vessels is elevated) or high cholesterol (when you have more of the waxy, fat-like substance in your blood than your body needs) may be passed down to you genetically. You can also inherit increased risks for heart disease based on your ethnicity. African-Americans, Mexican-Americans, and native Hawaiians are just a small sample of those who can inherit a greater risk for heart disease.

Your Age – An increased risk of cardiovascular disease as you age? That is probably the one risk of which everyone is keenly aware. Yet, that increased risk doesn't just magically appear once you reach the age of 65. In 2009, the Harvard Medical School reported as many as four percent to ten percent of all heart attacks occur before the age of 45.

The Risks You Can Reduce

Now, for some good news. Well, as good as news can be when it comes to talking about risk factors for heart disease and stroke. Many risk factors can be controlled and reduced enough to become more of an annoyance than a true risk factor.

High Cholesterol – Your body needs the cholesterol that flows through your blood. Unfortunately, if you have too much of the bad stuff (low-density lipoproteins or LDL) and not enough of the good stuff (high-density lipoproteins or HDL) that blood cholesterol can clog up your arteries, which can increase your risk for cardiovascular disease.

According to the CDC, more than 90 million U.S. adults age 20 or older have total cholesterol numbers higher than the recommended maximum of 200 mg/dL, and many of them don't even know it. For most people, high cholesterol is caused by an unhealthy diet, but some—myself included—have inherited a disfunction called familial hypercholesterolemia which can only be treated by medication.

While I will list many other risk factors that you should try and control with dietary changes and medication, high cholesterol is listed first because, according to Dr. Lawrence Liao, a board-certified cardiologist, the Framingham Risk Score—an algorithm used to assess your risk for heart disease—"gives more points to high cholesterol than the other factors, so if you can only change one thing, I would target that."

High Blood Pressure - Hypertension, more commonly known as high blood pressure, increases your heart's workload. This causes the heart's muscle to thicken, become stiffer, and function abnormally. It can increase your risk of a heart attack, stroke, and congestive heart failure, but with the right diet, exercise, monitoring, and medication, you can keep your blood pressure in line with the recommended 120 (systolic) over 80 (diastolic) maximum.

Diabetes – There are many forms of diabetes—Type 1, Type 2, Gestational, and even Prediabetes—but they all have one thing in common: you have too much sugar in your blood. Medication, diet, and exercise can all help control diabetes—a good thing as the American Heart Association reports those with high blood sugar are two to four times more likely to die from heart disease.

Stress – We all feel times of emotional or physical tension. Also known as stress. Not all stress is bad. It's just your body's way of protecting you and helping you push through a crisis or meet a tough deadline. However, when you face stress, your body responds by releasing a hormone called cortisol. A little cortisol is fine and normal. However, the University of Rochester Medical Center suggests that high, ongoing, levels of cortisol from stress can lead to increases in cholesterol, blood sugar, and blood pressure. And, as you have already read, each is a significant risk for cardiovascular disease.

Fortunately, you don't need to stress as much about stress as a risk for a heart attack or stroke. As you will explore in Chapter 8, stress can be reduced in several ways, including light exercise, yoga, and even breathing techniques.

Alcohol – "Really, even one glass of beer or wine is going to compromise my heart health?" I hear you ask. Please don't fret! Remember, we are talking about the risks we can reduce, and complete abstinence is not something many experts recommend when it comes to alcohol and heart disease. While many studies have suggested a positive link between drinking a moderate amount of red wine and good heart health, you should take into consideration your current alcohol consumption. If you don't drink alcohol, don't start. There are many better ways to optimize your heart. If you find yourself often pouring a whiskey or beer, then consider keeping to the guidelines suggested by the U.S. Department of Health and Human Services and U.S. Department of Agriculture, and limit your alcohol consumption to no more than two alcoholic drinks per day for men and no more than one alcoholic drink per day for women.

Obesity – Obesity is a chronic disease. According to a 2020 CDC data brief, obesity affects 42.4 percent of U.S. adults. Obesity can lead to high cholesterol, high blood pressure, and Type 2 diabetes—all risk factors for cardiovascular disease—but according to researchers at the University of Glasgow, obesity is a risk factor in its own right, with obese middle-aged men demonstrating a 60 percent increased risk of dying from a heart attack than those without obesity.

For many years the Body Mass Index (BMI) was the golden metric for calculating obesity, but it's now considered flawed by many. It merely looks at your height and weight and often neglects to take into account your muscle mass and other physical attributes. For example, there are many professional athletes and bodybuilders who are technically obese—try telling

Dwayne "The Rock" Johnson he's obese! Instead, when using diet and exercise to reduce obesity and associated cardiovascular disease risks, studies have shown that the average man should aim for a waist measurement of less than 40 inches and the average woman less than 35 inches.

The Risks You Can Eliminate

Lastly, there are some cardiovascular disease risk factors that you can look to eliminate from your daily life. I'm not suggesting you go cold turkey right away and some you may find impossible to ever reach total elimination. However, any good cardiologist will ask you to remove these risk factors from your life and I'm not about to sugar-coat this section. Sorry, but you need to accept that these need to go.

Smoking – Tobacco smoking is a major risk factor for a heart attack and stroke and causes one of every four deaths from cardiovascular disease. You've likely read the studies, seen the TV commercials, and heard stories of smokers that have died early, yet smoking is addictive and understandably hard to quit. My father-in-law used to smoke. He couldn't quit cold turkey, so he switched to chewing tobacco. After a few years, he then switched to Life Saver mints (now that's an appropriate candy name for a former smoker!). Today, he's in his seventies, still going strong, and tobacco-free. In Chapter

9, you'll learn more about the cardiovascular risks of smoking and tips for quitting.

Inactivity – Not getting your butt out of your chair and exercising is one of the biggest causes of cardiovascular disease. How so? Because, when you're inactive, you increase your likelihood of high cholesterol, high blood pressure, obesity, and a myriad of other heart disease and stroke risk factors. And this is not a risk factor you can brush off until you have plenty of free time in retirement. A 2014 study by the British Journal of Sports Medicine suggested that from the age of 30 until your late 80s, low physical activity had more negative influence than any other heart disease risk factor.

Fortunately, you don't need to be anxious about the possibility of later chapters recommending you become a professional athlete, run a marathon, or bench press 300 pounds. The *Physical Activity Guidelines for Americans,* 2nd edition, recommends you get just 150 minutes per week of moderate-intensity aerobic activity or 75 minutes if you engage in something more vigorous. The further good news? As you will learn in Part Three, that could simply mean taking a 25-minute brisk walk daily—which can even be split up throughout your day!

Unhealthy Foods – Wait? Am I about to suggest you eliminate ALL junk food? No, I'm not a registered dietician nor some fad-diet YouTube guru. However, many foods are just plain bad for you. And, the greater the number of contributing risk factors you have in your life, the greater the importance to eliminate as much unhealthy food as possible.

You'll learn more about eliminating cardiovascular-damaging foods in Chapter 9, but for now, just know that fast food, cooked in unhealthy fats, and smothered in salt can lead to high cholesterol, high blood pressure, obesity, and consequently, cardiovascular disease.

Ignorance is Not Bliss

Have you ever convinced yourself that you don't need to worry about testing for early signs of cardiovascular disease because you have no symptoms and you feel fine? Certainly, there are some scans and tests that are simply too impractical to have carried out. For example, having a CT (computerized tomography) scan or angiogram at the age of 40, when you have no symptoms of heart disease, just doesn't make practical or financial sense. However, checking your blood pressure can be done quickly with an automatic sphygmomanometer—also known as a blood pressure monitor. You can check your sugar levels with the prick of your finger and a blood glucose meter. And even your cholesterol numbers can be checked with a quick blood test at your doctor's office. Not knowing about any hidden risks for cardiovascular disease does not negate them.

Thankfully, I became aware that I had the inherited form of high cholesterol when I was in my late twenties. While having a routine eye exam, the optometrist noticed a milky-white ring around each of my eyes' iris. She let me know this was often a sign of high cholesterol and that I should have my doctor conduct a blood test. Sure enough, my cholesterol was in the high 300s and so I knew that I needed to mitigate that risk factor quickly with statin drugs.

Some risk factors are more obvious and manifest themselves early on. Others can be quickly checked and monitored from the comfort of your own home. And some can only be discovered by a medically qualified professional. And that's why, in Chapter 3, you'll learn why your doctor is going to be one of the most important allies in your quest to optimize your heart health.

Application

Make a note of any of the above risk factors you or a close family member have.

3

Doctors Really Do Know Best

It's not like you've never had a doctor's appointment before. You might even be one of the few people who enjoy the time spent discussing their health inside and out. Yet, you are forgiven if you have some degree of anxiety at the prospect of discussing your potential cardiovascular disease risk factors. After all, you don't want to have it confirmed that you have high cholesterol, elevated blood pressure, or obesity. I know I didn't.

While you will read later chapters that endeavor to help you optimize your heart through diet and exercise, if you acted on just one chapter in this book, it should be this one. Speaking to your doctor or health care provider is the most important initial step you can take to reduce your risk of a heart attack or stroke. Before I made changes to my diet and physical activity, I visited my doctor and discussed my concerns about my heart health, had my blood lipid panel updated, and talked through the plans my own personal trainer had designed for me. It was a crucial visit, eight months before my stroke.

With that in mind, the following is my best advice to you, learned from countless visits with my primary care physician (PCP), cardiologists, neurologists, and many other medical specialists. And, while I will share commonly held best practices for evaluating those at risk for heart disease or stroke, I am not a doctor, never played a doctor, and have never watched the television shows "Grey's Anatomy" or "The Good Doctor."

Checking You Inside and Out

If you did your assignment from Chapter 2, you should arrive at your doctor's office with your list of potential risk factors for cardiovascular disease. Your doctor should already have a record of the medications you take, any previous diagnoses made, and even notes about previous chats and vitals. Once they understand your reignited desire to optimize your heart, they will likely carry out some, if not all of the assessments below.

Height and weight – I'm not a fan of the BMI scale, but unless a doctor brings a tape measure to work each day and some calipers to take body fat measurements, it really is the fastest way for them to quickly assess your risk for obesity.

Pulse and blood pressure – A weak, fast, or erratic pulse are all warning signs that your doctor checks. They will also measure your blood pressure to look for systolic and diastolic readings that indicate hypertension (high blood pressure) and less common, hypotension (low blood pressure).

Heart sounds – When your doctor listens to your heart, they are primarily screening for any murmurs, irregular rhythms, or signs that any of your heart's valves are leaking. They also listen to both your heart and lungs for general signs of congestive heart failure.

Swelling – This one baffled me at first. Hello? My heart is not in my ankle? It's about as far away from my heart's location as possible! However, I've since learned that the distance from my heart to my ankles is a key reason why doctors will often check that location for any signs of swelling. Swelling can indicate poor blood circulation.

Electrocardiogram – A mouthful of a word often shortened to EKG or ECG. While it can look like something scary is about to happen, the electrodes they position on your chest are harmless. They simply let your doctor measure the electrical activity of your heart and can quickly identify a whole host of potential issues. Even more comforting than the fact that the test is painless is that it generally takes just seconds.

Blood test – If your doctor doesn't draw blood personally, you will likely still have it taken by a laboratory technician. While many different tests can be carried out on your blood, a lipid (fat) panel and glucose (sugar) levels are the ones you and your doctor will be the most interested in measuring.

Once your doctor has carried out an initial assessment, they may wait until they have your blood test results in hand before explicitly outlining a treatment plan for you. However, that won't stop them from making some preliminary recommendations for how you can improve your heart health. As you brace yourself for a possible list of new medications you will now need to take each day, you might be pleasantly surprised by the first steps your doctor suggests you undertake.

Optimize Your Lifestyle

While your doctor is indeed the one most likely to prescribe a statin to reduce your high cholesterol or a diuretic to control your hypertension, that is not always the first step they will recommend. "We usually recommend lifestyle optimization for all patients. Use of medicines then depends on how out of range the other things are," says Dr. Lawrence Liao. In other words, your doctor will want you to look at making changes to your diet and activity levels as a first step towards optimizing your heart health. If those lifestyle changes prove to be ineffective—or not quite effective enough—then they will probably start you out on the lowest dosage of the drug that has proven to be the most effective, with the least side effects, for your specific heart disease symptoms.

The sooner you talk to your doctor about your potential risks for cardiovascular disease, the earlier you can reduce those risks by making changes to your lifestyle. However, whether you procrastinated too long on lifestyle changes, didn't see a positive result from the new medications prescribed, or simply baffled your primary care physician with some kind of heart issue beyond their general level of care, you may find yourself being referred to a specialist: a cardiologist.

A Cardiologist Specializes in Your Heart

It's not that your family doctor doesn't personally want to help you with your heart optimization, it's just that they know when a condition is well beyond their generalized scope of medical care. If that condition is one that requires immediate attention, your doctor will likely have a referral relationship already in place with a trusted cardiologist. If your doctor tells you to see them this week—or perhaps the same day—then you should do so. Don't delay or second guess them.

That scenario certainly sounds scary, but let's be realists here. If you're speaking to your doctor because you've read this book and decided to take charge of your heart health before your heart health takes charge of you, then it's likely your need to speak to a cardiologist is not an urgent one. In such a case, you should still consider the cardiologist being recommended by your doctor. They know them well, likely have great channels of communication open to them, and there's a good chance they are already in-network with your medical insurance and maybe even part of the same medical practice.

That doesn't mean you can't shop around, though. I've often asked family and friends for their recommendations for a specialist doctor. I've conducted Google searches and read online reviews to find someone who I believe fits not just my heart health needs but also appears to match up with my personality preferences. I even once—and don't judge me on this—picked a cardiologist because, all else being equal, he graduated from the same school my wife and I support each football season. Go, Wolfpack!

Don't Be One and Done

Whether you're in the expert care of your general healthcare provider or under the watchful eye of a board-certified cardiologist, don't let this be a one-time interaction. It's vital that you check in with your doctor regularly. That doesn't mean you have to go visit them in person every month. You can give them a call. Use an online patient portal to send a question. Or conduct a telehealth—a virtual, online video—chat. Connect with them about any concerns, improvements, or changes in health as soon as they become evident.

Of course, there are some situations where there is no alternative to an in-office visit. Perhaps one of the most essential reasons to go back to see your doctor is to get your numbers checked. That can cover a host of different metrics—blood pressure, cholesterol levels, etc.—but often you will need to venture out to your doctor's office on whatever schedule they deem appropriate. A trip to your doctor's office can sometimes seem tedious, so why not make a game out of it?

Achieve a New Low Score

When you were a kid—or maybe you're still a kid at heart—you loved to achieve the highest possible score on video games. Don't deny it, you did. Even today, you may hope to achieve a new personal record for the most views, likes, or comments on a selfie you posted to social media. So, why not transfer that competitive spirit to your heart health numbers? I know I do, frequently. For example, my cholesterol was once as high as 353—when normal levels should be under 200. This is not the kind of high score anyone wants! Ever since, I have tried all manner of diets, exercises, and medications to try and reduce that number as low as I can. My genetic disorder meant I rarely saw a number below 200. So, when my cardiologist suggested I add Repatha injections to my cholesterol-reducing medications, you can bet I celebrated when my blood panel came back and showed a new low score of 97! Goal achieved!

Whether it's reducing your blood pressure, scaling back the number of medications you take, shrinking the number of inches on your waist, or running your fastest 5K, goals are an important part of anyone's journey to better heart health. The key is to set goals that are Specific, Measurable, Attainable, Relevant, and Timely. It's time to turn your heart health motivation into SMART goals.

Application

Make a list of questions you have for your doctor about your current heart health. Don't hold back; there are no dumb questions and your doctor is not afraid of what you've read on Google!

4

Turn Your Goals into Habits

There are three Stages of Change when it comes to modifying your behavior to improve your heart health. Now, before I share these with you, they are not the Transtheoretical Model of behavior change found in most psychology books—although, true story, I did study psychology in school for two years. No, these are three simple steps that I have personally experienced and have witnessed in others. When it comes to optimizing your heart health, you're likely already in Stage One of change: you found your motivation.

Stage One of Change: Motivation

Please remind me—and yourself—why did you decide to read this book? Perhaps you had a health scare. Maybe you have a wedding coming up—yours or one of your kid's—and want to look and feel fabulous!

Or, you are finally planning a dream vacation to Hawaii and want to be able to climb the incredibly steep and challenging stairway to the top of Diamond Head Crater. I am sure there are many reasons but, likely, the chief of which is that you finally found the motivation to reduce your risk of a heart attack or stroke.

For Gary Snow, an IT technician for a law enforcement agency, it was a realization that he had reached his highest weight of 304 pounds, had high blood pressure, high cholesterol, and even a fatty liver—all at the age of just 40. "My doctor told me that all my blood work indicated that I was not only morbidly obese but in severe danger of a heart attack," recalls Snow. "I had to make a change or else I would likely not live to see my kids finish school or get married."

Once Snow's motivation was revealed to him, he moved on to the next stage: setting a goal.

Stage Two of Change: Goals

Being motivated to get started is one thing, but if you don't have a goal to work towards, what's your initial direction? If you jumped in your car and went for a drive without setting a destination, you could end up back where you started. That said, if your final destination is Hollywood but you live in Manhattan, you shouldn't try to make the 2,800-mile trip in one sitting. You need to plan out shorter, achievable goals. "I think it's important to keep a goal in front of me. It helps keep me focused," says Snow.

Gary Snow started running races, from 5Ks to full marathons, to keep himself motivated towards better heart health. "My overarching goal, I think, is to continue to live healthy to be a good example to my children and those around me." Snow continues, "As far as immediate goals, I always try to keep a race in front of me. Having something to train for helps keep me focused."

When it comes to setting your short-term goals, the American Council on Exercise recommends the SMART method: **S**pecific, **M**easurable, **A**ttainable, **R**elevant, and **T**imely.

Specific – Don't be ambiguous with what you wish to accomplish. Don't just say, you want to "get healthy." Instead, be more specific with your goal, such as "I want to run a 5K race."

Measurable – Make sure your goal is something that can be easily measured. For example, don't set a goal to "improve my cholesterol numbers" when you can set something more measurable, such as "I want to reduce my LDL cholesterol by 30 points."

Attainable – Set a realistic goal. A good way to do that is to ask yourself, how attainable do I believe my goal is on a scale of 1 to 10? "I want to lose 20 pounds in one month" would probably score a 1 or a 2 out of 10, whereas "I want to lose 6 pounds over the next month" may be more achievable for you and thus score close to a 9 or 10.

Relevant – Running a race—of any distance—may not match up with your interests. You may have a knee injury that prevents you from even considering such a notion. Make sure your goal matches up with your motivation for optimizing your heart health. If you want to be able to go biking with your children, the goal of being able to cycle 10 miles in one outing is much more relevant.

Timely – Pick a timeline for any goal you set. Perhaps go as far as setting a timeline within a timeline. Anyone else recalling the movie "Inception" after that statement? If you want to lose 6 inches from your waist over the next 6 months, why not also set a goal of losing one inch each month?

Whatever goals you set for yourself, there will be one of two possible outcomes: failure or success. No one likes to talk about failure, but you may well find that you fail to achieve a goal that you set for yourself. And you know what? That's okay. Maybe something fun happened such as a family vacation or something life-changing such as losing your job. Whatever caused you to miss that goal shouldn't stop you from setting your next goal. You may have to lower your target or lengthen your timeline, but don't just give up. Remind yourself of your motivation and remember that you're working towards that destination, and that the goals along the way might just need a detour now and then.

If you succeed in achieving your goal, then you have two rewards coming your way. The first is something you decided on the day you set your goal. A new outfit, a day at the spa, or even the latest gadget. This is the reward that matched your mindset at the beginning of your journey. The second reward is one that you perhaps didn't even think about. For example, how much you enjoy the new healthy habits you have created for yourself.

Stage Three of Change: Habits

As you achieve the SMART goals you set for yourself, you may soon discover they become second nature to you. They are no longer deliberate goals you work towards but instead have become habits that work in you. How long will that take? I knew you were going to ask that, so I looked it up.

Like me, you've probably heard it takes 30 days for something new (good or bad) to become a habit. Actually, you may have heard all kinds of numbers, because there's no magic number of days that works for everyone. There is, however, one study published in the European Journal of Social Psychology that found it takes an average of 66 days to form a new habit. Whatever the magic number that works for you, let it be an encouragement. An encouragement that, if you miss a workout in the first week of your exercise goal or cave in and eat that delicious pepperoni pizza after eating healthy for 13 days straight, it's to be expected. You have months or even years of bad habits ingrained in you and those will take some time—maybe even more than 66 days—before they are fully replaced with healthier alternatives.

Don't give up! Gary Snow didn't.

"Just know that there are no shortcuts. The hardest part is taking that first step and keeping yourself determined to be a healthier you," encourages Snow. At last check, he has lost over 110 pounds in the last six years, and has run both the Boston and New York marathons.

Snow realized that, just like running a marathon, you often find even the most difficult journey is better when you use the help of others. "Surround yourself with a supportive network and lean on them when you need to." A support network of like-minded, encouraging people is a valuable structure to have in place when starting any journey to better health. In Chapter 5 you might just be surprised by the various types of support available to you.

Application

What's your first SMART goal? Give it some thought and get ready to create new healthy habits.

5

Your Support Network

A study by psychology professor Dr. Gail Matthews revealed that when you write down your goal, outline the plan you have in place to achieve it, send it to a supportive friend, and provide weekly updates, you are 33 percent more likely to achieve your goal than if you just kept a mental note of it and didn't tell anyone.

Whether you're the type of person who doesn't typically like to open up to others or the type who loves to share your entire life on social media, there are many different ways in which you can build your support group. This network will be a means for accountability and ultimately become a fan base that cheers for you as you take each small step towards your ultimate goal: an optimized heart!

Keep it Close

When looking to build your support network, start small and close to home. Your significant other is likely already supporting you when it comes to improving your heart health. They may even have been the one who bought this book for you! They should be the first person you ask for support, as teaming up with them can help you both improve your heart health. A study published by the JAMA Internal Medicine found that when one partner changed to a healthier behavior, the other partner was more likely to either quit smoking, increase physical activity, or experience five percent or more weight loss!

Perhaps you don't have a partner, or you feel you need more than just one other person's support. Where should you turn next? Ask your closest friends and family members if they would be willing to provide some emotional support and accountability. My wife and her sister often use each other for accountability and praise for their weekly weigh-ins while trying to lose a few pounds. The key to building your initial support group is to pick those that will provide the style of support that works best for your personality type:

> **Inspiring** – you love praise, inspiration, and encouragement
>
> **Practical** – you thrive on practical guidance, direction, and instruction

Emotional – you look for a shoulder to lean on, empathy, and understanding

Once you have a close-knit support group, that may well be all you need. But what if you need more help?

Local Support Groups

If you thrive in a group environment, then the support of just one or two individuals may not be enough for you. In this case, you can grow your network by either adding more family members, friends, and neighbors or look into other, local, in-person support groups.

Weight Watchers – Founded in 1963, Weight Watchers, now going by the simplified WW brand, has thousands of in-person and virtual workshop meetings around the world and is a great option for anyone needing accountability and support for both diet and exercise.

The YMCA – The YMCA is best known for its gyms, swimming pools, and exercise groups, but offers much more than that. With more than 2,700 locations covering over 10,000 communities, you may discover your local Y has many support groups, including Journey to Healthy Living which offers moderate physical activity, book discussions, food education, and journaling within a supportive environment.

Local Hospitals – You may have noticed your local hospital rebranding itself to include "wellness" or "health" in its name. As more local hospitals focus resources on preventative health services, you will likely find a local group that meets to provide support for weight loss, heart health, diabetes, and more.

Meetup – While Meetup is an online platform, its main focus is to help people "meetup" offline and has hundreds of thousands of local group listings. Running, yoga, cooking classes, smoking cessation, and weight loss can all be found on Meetup.com, but don't just stop there! Create a Meetup listing and build your own support group, for your zip code, with similar risk factors, and common goals.

American Heart Association – Your local chapter of the American Heart Association, AHA, is a great place to look for local groups designed to inspire and motivate you towards optimizing your heart. Join a heart-healthy cooking class or find a local walking group. The AHA has partnerships all over the country and can help you find a group that will meet your goals.

If the thought of meeting real people, in real life, gives you sweaty palms, don't worry. There are plenty of alternative platforms and channels for building your support network.

Digital Accountability

The World Wide Web is something I use for my own heart optimization accountability. As someone who has spent more than two decades focusing on internet marketing, you can bet that when a friend started an online accountability and encouragement group named Marketing Fitness and asked me to join, I didn't pass up the opportunity. If you already enjoy connecting with others online, there are many different support options you can explore.

Facebook – While not the first social network, Facebook is the one where you will most likely find many of your existing friends while also making new ones. Facebook Pages are a great channel for following a health expert to receive their advice while also keeping connected by leaving comments or sharing to their wall. Facebook Groups are an even better way to connect with others and get support and accountability. Often marked private—so only members can see the posts—Groups let you share your successes and failures and get the support of others. And you'll find Facebook Groups as broadly organized as Weight Loss Motivation or as small and niche as Women with Heart Failure, Cardiomyopathy and other heart conditions!

MyFitnessPal – I have used MyFitnessPal many times over the past decade or so. Since its launch in 2005, the online website and smartphone app has grown to over 150 million users, and for good reason. It provides so many different levels of accountability and support. You can start by simply tracking your diet and exercise goals privately. When you add friends and contacts, you can decide what information is shared with them and let them comment and like your workouts and food diary entries. MyFitnessPal also has a very active forum where you can share goals, receive encouragement, or set new challenges with others.

Strava – There are many different fitness apps out there, but Strava is my personal favorite, so it's the one I will recommend for those looking for a different kind of accountability and motivation: competitiveness. Now, that works in a couple of different ways. Primarily, I use Strava to track my workouts, my runs, and my bike rides. It offers so much analytical data and lets you see how each effort compares to your previous one. Heart rate, cadence, time, calories burned; you name it. It also keeps track of your week over week performance so you can see if you've slacked off recently. Self-motivation and accountability from one app!

Even better, Strava lets you add connections—friends or strangers—and help each other to stay motivated. You can each give the other's physical activity a kudos thumbs-up or leave an encouraging comment. You may even find yourself fired up by your friend's efforts and try to better them!

Lastly, Strava offers groups that let you connect with those with similar interests, health challenges, or goals. I belong to the Running With Asthma group, and getting kudos from another runner, half-way around the world, is a great way to keep me motivated to optimize my heart.

Garmin – I almost went with Smartwatch for this subheading because I know many friends love their Fitbit or Apple Watch, but I decided to stick with something that I personally use and love: Garmin. A Garmin smartwatch will help you stick to just about any fitness goal you have set for yourself. It tracks just about everything. Yes, walking, running, biking, weightlifting, and swimming, but it also tracks other exercises, too—and you can even customize it to track your Zumba class or ballroom dancing.

In addition, you can monitor your sleep patterns, your heart rate, your blood oxygen levels, and even your stress! You can share stats with your friends or join a group of others that share your health goals and also happen to wear a Garmin watch. So, yes, I am a Garmin fan, but write down exactly what type of tracking, support, and accountability you want from a smartwatch and pick the one that will best help you achieve your goals.

There are so many different digital devices and online platforms you can use to build a large support group, but if, after reading through all my suggestions, you still consider yourself someone who does better when they go it alone, there's no need to expose your challenges, your achievements, and your goals to others.

Be Your Own Biggest Fan

As someone labeled Generation X, I consider myself as having one foot in the Millennial camp that loves the internet and the latest gadgets, while the other foot is in camp Baby Boomer that lovingly clings to pens, paper, and privacy. I often experience the world through both lenses. That is why the last recommendation for accountability and support is more venerable, tangible, and private: write it down and keep yourself accountable. Yes, sharing your goals and your progress with others has shown to be the most effective way to stay accountable. However, if doing so creates anxiety or makes you feel too self-conscious, then you risk sabotaging your goals.

Instead, keep a private journal and set a goal that comes with a reward that you'll give yourself. You may write that you will get a pedicure if you lose five pounds. Or jot down you get to buy a new fishing pole if you go two weeks without a cigarette. The key is to set a reward that you forfeit if you don't achieve your goal. Why? Because a study by the Perelman School of Medicine at the University of Pennsylvania found that those who risked losing a reward set for a goal achieved their goal 50 percent more of the time than those who had no reward to lose.

Don't Sweat It Just Yet

Over the previous five chapters, you've read about the importance of improving your heart health, understanding your cardiovascular risk factors, speaking to your doctor, and turning your motivation into goals first, and then habits. Now that you have an idea of how to set for yourself accountability, support, and encouragement, you may be ready to hit the gym or start racking up your daily steps. While exercise is a critical component for optimizing your heart health, there are four equally important areas that you can look to first, without perspiring a single bead of sweat. The second part of *Optimize Your Heart* begins with optimizing your diet.

Application

Think about what type of support you need to achieve your goals. Pick from any of the above or head to Google and search for an app, local group, or device that stands out as a great fit for you.

Part Two: Your Wellness Comes First

6

Eat, Drink, and Be Healthy

Abs are made in the kitchen. You can't outrun a bad diet. It takes five minutes to eat 500 calories, but two hours to burn them off. Any of these statements sound familiar? Even if they are new to you, they all share a common theme that's important for anyone looking to lose weight, feel energized, and lower the risks for cardiovascular disease: optimize your diet.

There's a very good reason why this chapter is prioritized before chapters that discuss sleep, stress reduction, kicking bad habits, or even exercise. What you eat and drink each day is the most important self-improvement you can make to optimize your heart and reduce your chances of having a stroke or heart attack.

Millions of guides have been written about diets and healthy eating, so I am not about to pretend that I am a qualified dietician or experienced nutritionist by mapping out exactly what you need to add or remove from your diet. However, it doesn't have to be that complicated and precise, anyway. You just need to know a few basics of nutrition.

Simple Caloric Math

I hated math in school. I never was much good at solving complex mathematic formulas. However, when it comes to fueling your body, the math is pretty simple. When you provide your body with the exact number of calories it burns each day, you will neither gain nor lose weight. If you need to gain weight, you need to be in a calorie surplus. If you are trying to lose weight, you need to be in a calorie deficit. Simple enough, right? Well, it is, as long as you know how many calories your body needs each day.

It wasn't until I started tracking my diet and exercise that I heard of these three little letters: BMR. At first, I thought it was a typo for BMI, Body Mass Index, which many professionals use to determine if you are underweight, normal, overweight, or obese. I was wrong. BMR is real and it means Basal Metabolic Rate. BMR is the number of calories your body burns each 24-hour cycle when not doing any physical activity. Conduct a Google search for "BMR calculator" and you will find dozens of free tools that collect your weight, height, age, and sex and provide a rough calculation of your BMR.

Once you have that number, you'll have a good idea of how many calories your body needs each day.

However, it's not enough to simply know how many calories your body needs. You also need to know the main nutrients that make up your daily caloric intake.

A Micro Look at Macronutrients

You've probably heard of the term macronutrients, often shortened to macros, and may even be able to quickly recall them. But, in case you need a refresher, or just want to test my knowledge, allow me to explain the three essential nutrients that provide your body with calories.

Carbohydrates – Carbohydrates, frequently referred to as carbs, are your body's main source of energy and provide important fuel. They come in both healthy, complex carbs from foods such as fruits, vegetables, and whole grains, and unhealthy, refined carbs such as sugar-sweetened beverages, candy, cookies, and white bread.

Proteins – Proteins are the building blocks used by your body to grow muscle, repair tissue, and maintain a healthy immune system. Protein-rich foods include meat, chicken, fish, eggs, dairy, nuts, and tofu. If you hear the expression "lean protein," that just means the protein is coming from a source that is also lower in saturated fats and cholesterol.

Fats – Fats often get a bad rap but are as vital to your body as the other two macros. They provide you with energy and support cell growth. They also help your body to absorb some vitamins and produce important hormones. Fats provide more energy per gram than proteins or carbs and can be found in meats, dairy, oils, and nuts. There are four different types of fats. The healthier kinds are monounsaturated and polyunsaturated fats, while the unhealthy kinds are saturated and trans-unsaturated fatty acids, also known as trans fats.

If you're hoping I am going to share a magic formula to help you calculate your macros and lose weight, gain muscle, and feel fabulous, I'm sorry to disappoint you. As a reminder, you are wonderfully and beautifully unique. A registered dietitian nutritionist who specializes in heart health is the person to speak with should you wish to know what percentage each macro should make up of your daily diet. However, a good, if not generalized, place to start is the United States Department of Agriculture guideline: 45 to 65 percent carbs, 10 to 35 percent protein, 20 to 35 percent fat.

The Unsung Macro Heroes

Did you already know the three core macronutrients essential for your body? Great job! Your gold star is in the mail. But, do you know the two unsung macro heroes that are equally essential for your heart health? No peeking ahead! Any guess? Okay, you can peek.

Water and fiber.

Of course, you have heard of water and fiber, but did you know that these are widely considered to be macronutrients, too? The reason why they often don't get listed alongside proteins, carbs, and fats is that they do not provide any nutritional value. Yet, both are vital to your body!

H2 Oh Yeah!

Water is essential to your body in so many different ways. Water is a delivery mechanism for vitamins and nutrients, it helps flush out toxins and waste, and regulates your body's temperature and metabolism. The problem is, you may not be drinking enough water each day.

There are many different studies and guidelines about how much water the average person should drink each day, but don't consider yourself average. Instead, consume enough water each day—drink it or eat water-rich foods—that your urine looks closer in color to lemonade than apple juice. Why? Your urine contains the chemical urobilin which is the primary source of its yellow coloring. The more hydrated you are the higher percentage of water to urobilin in your urine. When you are too dehydrated, your urine has a higher percentage of urobilin and thus looks darker yellow, or even orange, in color. And now you will always be fascinated by the color of your pee-pee.

The Power of Fiber

While fiber is technically just a type of carbohydrate—one that your body cannot digest—I like to consider it a separate macro because it plays such a vital role in your body. Fiber not only improves digestion and blood sugar regulation, it also has many heart health benefits, too! A study led by Dr. Cheryl R. Clark found that diets high in fiber may help reduce your risk of developing diabetes, heart disease, and stroke.

Lindsey Pine, a registered dietitian nutritionist and author of *Mediterranean Diet Meal Prep Cookbook* became a huge fan of fiber after her husband suffered a stroke at the age of 41 and was later diagnosed with heart failure. She recommends fiber-rich foods such as fruits, vegetables, whole grains, nuts, and seeds. "Foods with fiber have amazing heart-healthy nutrients such as vitamins, minerals, antioxidants, and phytochemicals," explains Pine. "I am definitely a believer in the power of fiber!"

Micronutrients Are Massively Important

You just read an important summary of macronutrients and the benefits to your body, but they are not the only nutrients that play a key role in optimizing your heart. Micronutrients—why are macronutrients often called macros yet rarely do I see the word "micros" used?—are primarily vitamins and minerals. They include vitamins A, B, C, D, E, K, and iron, selenium, zinc, and more.

How many of each do you need in a healthy diet? While there are recommended daily amounts, studies are mixed on how micronutrients affect your heart health. Many studies point to a deficiency in micronutrients leading to the development of cardiovascular disease, yet results are mixed as to whether vitamin and mineral supplements help improve your heart health. The best rule of thumb is to try and get as many vitamins and minerals from nutrient-rich foods and use supplements as a backup plan. Supplements may not significantly help, but they're cheap, easy, and worth trying. Just be sure to check with your medical provider first.

Eat the Food Your Heart Desires

Unless you read that subheading carefully, you might think I'm about to recommend a diet that includes all the pizza, fries, ice-cream, and beer you could ever want. That would be your "heart's desire," an idiom for your emotional needs, not what your physical heart desires. A subtle, but important, difference.

Your heart wants your daily caloric intake to incorporate as many fruits, veggies, whole grains, lean protein, and low-fat dairy as you can, literally, stomach.

At the same time reduce the amount of saturated fats, sugar-sweetened drinks, and sodium you consume. If you need direction for changing your eating habits, a good place to start is the DASH diet, which stands for **D**ietary **A**pproaches to **S**top **H**ypertension. Consistently ranked as one of the best out of more than 40 different diets in the world, the DASH diet was also ranked the Best Heart-Healthy Diet in the 2018 U.S. News & World Report's "Best Diets" rankings. Impressive!

Just as I would tell any client, the DASH diet is the best recommendation I can give you, but I understand that while it may be the perfect diet for your heart, it may not be one that you can adhere to. If you feel intimidated by the DASH diet, and when using a scale of 1 to 10 to measure your confidence in being able to stick with it, you score a low number, then I have a suggestion. Start with small changes first.

Sow the Seeds of Change

When I first changed my diet, I didn't just go on a diet. I found them too overwhelming and quite tasteless. My tongue and brain had been used to delicious comfort foods for the better part of 40 years. Switching to a DASH diet overnight was going to set me up for failure, not success. Instead, I started with small changes to my diet. Whole wheat wraps instead of white bread. Veggies instead of fries. I even—dare I admit this as someone who lives in the South?—switched from sweet tea to unsweet tea. Mercy!

When I asked Lindsey Pine about this, I was thankful to hear that I had taken the best approach for switching to a heart-healthy diet. "You're not destined to eat a boring, bland diet if you're eating for heart health," says Pine. "Make one change, conquer it, then move on to the next change to add on to your new healthier lifestyle." She suggests slowly adding more vegetables, berries, and omega-3 rich foods such as salmon, nuts, and seeds. The good news is you don't have to completely eliminate the tasty indulgences from your diet. "You can still eat treats. It's about balancing those healthy foods with treats," encourages Pine.

Okay, that was a pretty intense chapter to digest. Pun intended. After spending all that time focusing on macros, micros, and healthy eating, you could probably use a nap. Before you do, you may want to take a look at the next chapter.

Application

Use an online calculator to determine your BMR. Visit Heart.org for some heart-healthy recipes or speak to a registered dietician nutritionist who specializes in heart health.

7

Sleep Soothes Your Heart

There are a lot of recommendations in this book designed to help you optimize your heart health and reduce your risk of cardiovascular disease. See your doctor, change your diet, drink less alcohol, exercise more. I know it can all be a little overwhelming, but here's a recommendation that I hope you'll find easy to embrace: get enough sleep!

I regularly analyze the smorgasbord of stats provided by my smartwatch. Monitoring how much I sleep each night is vitally important if I am to reduce my likelihood of ever having another heart attack or stroke. When you sleep, your body regenerates tissue, lowers stress, improves mood, stores memories, and improves your immune function. And you don't have to do anything! Other than making sure you get enough quality sleep every 24 hours.

How Much Sleep is Enough?

According to the CDC, if you consistently sleep seven hours or more each night, you reduce your risk for a heart attack, stroke, coronary heart disease, diabetes, and many other chronic health conditions. That sounds like a no-brainer, right? Yet, the CDC also reports that one in three U.S. adults do not get enough sleep.

Not getting enough sleep doesn't just mean you feel sleepier and more sluggish as you make your way through the day, it can also result in you being less physically active and more likely to suffer from obesity. This is proven by the Nurses' Health Study which followed 60,000 women for 16 years and found those who slept five hours or less each night had a 30 percent higher risk of gaining 30 pounds throughout the study. That makes sense, right? The more time you are awake, the more opportunities you have to pass by your fridge or pantry and have a "snackcident." *<insert your groan here>*

Humor aside, physiology provides a clear reason as to why not getting enough sleep can lead to weight gain. A study published in the research journal Obesity found that if you don't get enough sleep you are more likely to have increased levels of a hunger hormone called ghrelin—often nicknamed Gremlin as it's mischievous and messes with your body! Ghrelin is more commonly known as the hunger hormone because it stimulates your appetite, increases your food intake, and promotes fat storage.

Lack of sleep can also cause your body to have decreased levels of the satiety hormone called leptin. Leptin sends signals to your brain that you have enough energy stored in your fat cells so there's no need to eat more.

If you're already getting seven or more hours of sleep each night and feel pretty refreshed each morning, then you can probably just skip to the next chapter—how often will an author suggest that? However, if you know you don't always hit that magic seven number, read on.

Get More ZZZZs

I just conducted a search for "get more sleep" on Amazon and there are over 1,000 books on the topic, so if you are truly struggling to get enough sleep, you should probably read a book that focuses on that topic or go speak to your doctor. However, these are some general tips to help you sleep the recommended seven hours or more.

Exercise more – When you exercise, your body needs more time to recover and rebuild. The National Sleep Foundation examined the relationship between sleep and exercise and found that you are more likely to sleep better if you exercise. And when researchers looked at 34 different studies that combined sleep with exercise, they found that "middle-aged and elderly adults" who exercised "increased sleep efficiency and duration regardless of the mode and intensity of activity, especially in populations suffering from disease."

Consume less caffeine – This tip might not work for everyone, but in general, try not to consume caffeine too close to your normal bedtime. Not only is caffeine a stimulant that can keep you awake at night, it's also a diuretic. That's a scientific term for I had to get up to pee three times last night!

Less screen time before bedtime – Most TVs, smartphones, and laptops emit a short-wavelength, artificial blue light which The National Sleep Foundation reports can mess with your body's internal clock, also known as your circadian rhythm, suppress the release of the sleep-inducing hormone called melatonin, and thus make it harder for you to fall asleep. Try to avoid screen time at least 30 minutes before you go to bed or look for a device or app that reduces the display's blue light once the sun sets.

Improve your sleep hygiene – You practice great body hygiene (I hope), so why not great sleep hygiene? Sleep hygiene involves using daily habits to get your body ready for a good night's sleep. For example, try to go to bed the same time each night, set your home's thermostat between 60 and 67 degrees, and play a soothing song to help you drift off. Musician and composer Jean-Michel Jarre's 47-minute "Waiting for

Cousteau" electronic lullaby usually sends me and my wife off to sleep every night!

This is not an exhaustive list of tips. You may find essential oils, herbal remedies, or a glass of warm milk at bedtime are also great options for you.

To Nap or Not to Nap, That is the Question

I have never been one to take a nap. I just can't fall off to sleep during the day. Yet, I know many others who can take a 20-minute siesta in the middle of the day. If you're having trouble getting in seven or more hours of sleep each night—perhaps due to work or a newborn baby—then studies have shown that taking a daytime nap "can" be beneficial.

I emphasize "can" because taking a daytime nap can be both good and bad for your heart health. If you are taking a nap out of choice because you know it will re-energize you and get you through the day, then a study published in the 2007 Archives of Internal Medicine suggests that you have a 37 percent lower risk of dying from heart disease, likely due to reduced cardiovascular stress offered by daytime sleep. Conversely, if you are sleeping during the day because you can't stay awake and know you are not sleeping well at night, then it could be due to sleep apnea, anemia, or some other underlying health issue. If you think that might be the case, then it's time to go back to your doctor.

Not Enough Might Be Enough

You are unique! So is your body's sleep needs and pattern. While seven or more hours is the generally accepted guideline for most adults, you might be the exception. Heck, even Buddy the Elf thrived on a full 40 minutes!

If you wake up feeling refreshed, get through your day without feeling sleepy, and can drink coffee and read your phone while propped up on your pillow at 2 a.m., then, you may well be getting all the sleep you need to ensure a healthy heart. There's no need to get stressed out just because you're not getting the recommended amount of sleep. Oh, and speaking of not getting stressed out...

Application

Track your sleep to see how much you are getting each night and note how you feel the following day.

8

Don't Stress Out

Have you ever felt so stressed that you just want to Hulk-smash something? The bad driver in front of you. The email inbox that never stops growing. Or, Loki for leading an alien invasion through a wormhole? That last one might not be a cause of stress for you, but you probably experienced at least one kind of stressful situation over the past month. The good news is that you are not alone. A 2017 American Psychological Association survey found that a whopping 80 percent of respondents reported experiencing at least one symptom of stress over the course of a month.

Even better news is that feeling stressed is normal. When stressed, your body responds by releasing cortisol and adrenaline hormones. This fight or flight response pumps extra blood to your muscles for immediate reaction, while also increasing your strength, heart rate, and blood pressure. Great for running away from a snake; bad if you're stuck at your office desk.

The downside is that frequent stress is unhealthy. Continual stress results in a buildup of cortisol in your body. A 2010 study published in the Journal of Clinical Endocrinology & Metabolism found high levels of cortisol strongly predict cardiovascular death among both persons with and without pre-existing cardiovascular disease. Those with the highest levels of cortisol were five times more likely to die of heart disease.

If this is all true, why haven't you heard of a drug that can quickly reduce the amount of cortisol in your body? It would fly off the pharmacist's shelves! The reason being is there is no concrete evidence that reducing high levels of cortisol will reduce your risk for a heart attack or stroke. In other words, you need to look for ways to reduce the amount of stress in your life and thus prevent your cortisol levels from being too high for too long in the first place.

"Reduce the amount of stress in my life? Got it!" I hear you thinking out loud. "I'll add Jack Daniels, Ben & Jerry, and Little Debbie to my heart health support group!" Sure, why not. In moderation. But turning to alcohol, ice cream, and cakes is not healthy, nor an effective way to reduce the amount of stress in your life. If you want to prevent high cortisol levels from increasing your risk for a stroke or heart attack, there are a variety of stress reduction methods to consider.

Actively De-stress

There are many activities and hobbies you can use to improve your overall heart health, but some are particularly beneficial in reducing stress.

Yoga – Yoga is a combination of physical, mental, and spiritual practices that originate in ancient India. Yoga in the western world combines physical postures (asanas), breathing techniques, and relaxation. "Asana is the physical practice of yoga whereby we connect breath, heart, mind, and body," explains Lisa O'Rear, a certified yoga instructor.

O'Rear suffered a stroke at the age of 34 and now uses yoga daily to improve her heart health. And science is on her side. A 2005 study published in the Medical Science Monitor showed that yoga can reduce your cortisol levels, stress, anxiety, and depression. Other studies have shown that yoga can also reduce your blood pressure, lower your LDL cholesterol, and even slow the progression of heart disease.

Massage – A massage is the manipulation of your body's soft tissue and muscles to increase the flow of blood and oxygen, decrease pain, and reduce stress. Bonnie Timan, a nationally certified massage therapist for over 20 years, has seen "hands-on" evidence (yay, for puns!) that a massage can help reduce cardiovascular disease risks. Timan explains, "A massage can help you reduce blood pressure, increase circulation, improve your mental performance, and enjoy deeper sleep."

Many studies have shown that a massage can improve your heart health and reduce your risk of cardiovascular disease.

Tai Chi – From my own experience, the ancient Chinese art of tai chi is much like yoga but is more dance-like in its form. Often combined with another ancient Chinese practice called qigong, both offer a great way to incorporate low-impact, flowy exercise into your life while also reducing stress. A Harvard Medical School study found tai chi also improves the quality of life for heart failure patients.

Light Exercise – The reason I list this beneficial activity as light exercise is that even with exercise, you can have too much of a good thing. A 2008 study published in the Journal of Endocrinological Investigation observed that moderate to high-intensity exercise provokes increases in circulating cortisol levels; whereas, low-intensity exercise resulted in a reduction in cortisol levels. Walking, dancing, swimming, and housework are all examples of light exercise. Unless housework stresses you out, in which case, don't do it and use "I need to reduce my cortisol levels" as your excuse.

Pets – Playing a game, stroking its fur, or enjoying the attention you get when returning from a hard day at the office are just some of the many cardiovascular benefits of owning a pet. Are you a cat person or a dog person? It doesn't matter. A 2019 study by Washington State University found that just ten minutes of interaction with a cat or dog significantly reduced the amount of cortisol in your body. And stress reduction doesn't just apply to pets of the fluffy kind. After all, how many times have you seen a fish tank at your dentist's office? Stress reduction can have fins, too!

Distract Yourself

Distracting your mind from the stress that has engulfed you can be a great way to prevent a high elevation of cortisol levels in your body.

Play a Game – Video games, board games, card games, or puzzles. Playing any kind of game can help distract you from life's stresses and improve your mood. A 2017 study published by the Human Factors and Ergonomics Society found that just five minutes of casual video gaming improved the mood and reduced the amount of workplace stress in participants.

Listen to Music – Actively listening to the type of music you love will help reduce the amount of stress in your body. You might enjoy the calming effect of instrumental or classical music. You may be the kind of person who loves to do hairbrush karaoke to your favorite Top 40 hit. Or, maybe your spouse loves to sing "Jeremiah was a bullfrog" at the top of their lungs while taking a stress-relieving hot shower. Okay, that last one may only apply to my wife.

Read a Book – Reading can be a healthy escape from the stress in your life. Whether you like the tactile feel of a paperback or prefer the convenience of an e-reader, reading your favorite book is good for your heart health. A 2009 study at the University of Sussex found that reading can reduce stress by up to 68 percent!

Laugh – I hope that *Optimize Your Heart* has already made you literally LOL at least once. I love humor and always look for it in every situation. Whenever you feel stressed, watching a TV comedy, listening to a funny podcast, or following funny memes on social media can all help reduce the amount of cortisol that builds up during tough times. And, I just have to include mention of this 2016 study Salivary Cortisol Levels: The Importance of Clown Doctors to Reduce Stress, where hospitalized children, who were entertained by clowns, showed a decrease in the amount of cortisol in their body. That's it! I want to become a clown doctor!

Be Still

Even if you can only find two minutes to try something—anything—to reduce the stress you are enduring, try these techniques.

Breathing – Sometimes we just need to focus on our breathing to reduce our stress levels. Lisa O'Rear explains the importance of conscious breathing. "Our unconscious breathing patterns are often tense, labored and at times can be erratic. When we practice long, smooth inhales and exhales, we support the parasympathetic nervous system reducing stress and its effects on the body and mind."

Here's a breathing technique that might help you. Breathe in, through your nose, slowly for a count of four. Hold that breath for a count of four. Then breathe out through your mouth for another count of four. Then wait four more seconds before starting over. If Navy Seals can use a similar method to calm themselves in combat, then you know this simple breathing technique can help lower your stress.

Prayer & Meditation – Spending time with God, or with your inner self, is a great way to block out the stress in your life and find peace. Prayer was the most important part of my stroke recovery and is key to Lisa O'Rear's heart health, too. "Prayer and a relationship with God is what keeps me going," explains O'Rear. "I survived my stroke because God is merciful and gracious. I do my best to cast all my doubts, worries, and fears upon Him."

Heart health benefits also come from using meditation to help clear your mind at times of stress. A meta-analysis study led by Maxwell V. Rainforth, Ph.D. in 2007 found that meditation helped reduce stress, blood pressure, and lowered the risk of cardiovascular death by 30 percent.

Phone a friend – When you feel stressed, it might be a good time to tap into the support network you built in Chapter 5. Send an email, call, text, or even video chat with your sibling, bestie, or favorite co-worker. Now's also a good time to learn an important adage that you should use when someone contacts you because they just need to vent and destress: Hear me now, listen to me later. In times of stress, we don't always need advice, just a shoulder to lean on.

Take a nap – In Chapter 7, you learned the potential heart health benefits of taking a nap. Just in case you need another excuse to take a siesta during the day, a 2015 study published in The Journal of Clinical Endocrinology and Metabolism found that after a bad night of sleep, a 30-minute nap can stop your stress hormones from increasing. Naptime!

These are just a few healthy ways you can reduce the amount of stress in your life and help prevent a heart attack or stroke. Give them a try and you may find one or two that become healthy habits after just 66 days. Not only will they reduce the amount of cortisol in your body, they may well become a replacement for any bad habits that can so easily wreck your heart health. Some you may already avoid, others you might struggle with, but they may be news to you.

Application

Pick one of the stress reduction methods listed and try it the next time you feel yourself turning green.

9

Breaking Bad Habits

In Chapter 2, you learned about the different risk factors that increase the likelihood of you having a heart attack or stroke. As a refresher, some can't be changed—your age, your gender, your heritage; some you can reduce—cholesterol, blood pressure, alcohol—but others "should" be eliminated. Tobacco smoking. Unhealthy foods. Inactivity.

Once again, you may notice I have emphasized an important verb: "should." I have been working with clients in many different capacities over the past 25 years and I always tell them the same thing: I will give you my best advice, but I understand that it's not always possible to follow my recommendations 100 percent, so do the best you can and modify where needed. That advice applies to this chapter. You absolutely should try to eliminate each of these bad habits as part of your effort to improve your heart health, but even if you just reduced the presence of each, you will feel better and likely reduce your risks of cardiovascular disease. Aim for the stars but celebrate even if you only reach the moon! You'll have still made a lot of progress!

Don't Inhale the Toxic Stuff

Whether you are a smoker or not, you already know that tobacco smoking is bad for you. Just as Jesus once said, "Let he who is without sin cast the first stone," I am not going to wag a finger, grab a soapbox, or mount a high horse and chastise you if you smoke. At least not until I can, hand-on-heart, say that my own diet, exercise, sleep, alcohol consumption, and urine color are as perfect as perfect can be. That said—sorry, but you knew this was coming—if you smoke, you should know just how great your risk is for a heart attack or stroke. Even if you don't smoke, you may know someone who does or perhaps even someone in your household smokes around you. They need to know, too!

According to the American Heart Association, smoking increases your risk of heart disease or stroke by two to four times. Men who smoke fewer than 11 cigarettes a day are still 46 percent more likely to have a stroke, while those who smoke 40 or more cigarettes a day are 556 percent more likely. Five hundred and fifty-six percent! Just when you thought I couldn't share any worse stat than that, women who smoke have a 25 percent higher risk of developing heart disease compared to men who smoke.

So, why is smoking bad for your heart health? Is it the addictive nicotine found in every cigarette or the tobacco smoke that raises your risk for heart disease? Both! While debates continue about whether nicotine itself is any more harmful than caffeine, it does raise your heart rate and your blood pressure while being far more addictive than even a triple espresso with an extra shot of espresso. Nicotine is also the main reason why people have trouble giving up smoking and thus continually pump their lungs, and their entire body, with tobacco smoke.

Cigarette smoke contains thousands of chemical components, including hundreds that are harmful to your health. According to the CDC, smoking has been shown to:

- Make your blood sticky and more likely to clot, a leading cause of heart attacks and strokes.
- Raise your triglycerides (a type of fat in your blood).
- Lower your "good" cholesterol (HDL).
- Cause thickening and narrowing of blood vessels.
- Increase the buildup of plaque (fat, cholesterol, and calcium) in your blood vessels.

So, how can you quit smoking?

I don't smoke, so I have no personal experience to pass on, but I do know many people who have successfully kicked the habit. Some have indeed gone cold turkey but others have found the following to be invaluable in their efforts to quit:

- Smoking cessation programs can often be found at your local hospital, doctor's office, or even your workplace.
- Nicotine replacement therapy, such as chewing gum, lozenges, patches, and sprays, can help you transition through the first few weeks of quitting.
- Your doctor may prescribe a medication designed to help curb your smoking withdrawal symptoms.
- While E-cigarettes are marginally healthier than cigarette smoking, vaping still fills your body with nicotine and cancer-causing chemicals and so should be a last resort when trying to quit.
- For more suggestions and guidance visit www.smokefree.gov or www.heart.org.

Quitting smoking is tough. Dying from smoking is tougher. The good news is that, after just one year of quitting, your risk for coronary heart disease is reduced by 50 percent. If you give your body 15 years of a smoke-free life, your risk for heart disease drops to that of a non-smoker. In other words, the sooner you quit, the longer you may live.

Don't Eat the Bad Stuff

There are lots of healthy foods you should add to your diet to optimize your heart. Fruits, vegetables, whole grains, nuts, and beans. There are also many foods that you should try to reduce. Processed meats, refined sugars, and white bread. However, if you want to turn the dial all the way to 11 on your healthy diet, there are two nutritional saboteurs that you should try to eliminate: unhealthy fats and excess sodium.

Unhealthy Fats – There are four types of fats and they are divided into two distinct groups. The healthy ones are monounsaturated and polyunsaturated fats. Unhealthy fats are saturated and trans-unsaturated fatty acids, known as trans fats.

Saturated fats can be found in foods like butter, palm and coconut oils, cheese, and even red meats. Eating foods with saturated fats can raise the levels of bad cholesterol in your blood and increase your risk for a heart attack or stroke.

Trans fats are like the evil twin sibling of an already evil person. These artificially created fats can raise your bad cholesterol, lower your good cholesterol, and increase your risk for cardiovascular disease. They are so bad for your heart health that the Food and Drug Administration has already taken steps to stop manufacturers from adding them to foods and beverages.

Eliminating both of these fats entirely from your diet is going to be virtually impossible. Some will still sneak through. That shouldn't stop you from always being on the lookout for saturated and trans fats in the foods that tempt you. Check the labels of packaged foods for ingredients such as partially hydrogenated oils or, when tempted by fast food, check the restaurant's website, or email them, and ask what type of cooking oil they use. For example, Chick-fil-A uses peanut oil. Peanut oil is one of the healthiest oils used by a fast-food chain. It is a vegetable oil that is naturally trans-fat-free, cholesterol-free, and low in saturated fats!

Excess Sodium – Sodium is an essential electrolyte that your body uses for proper nerve and muscle function. Your body only needs around 500 milligrams of sodium each day, yet the average American consumes 3,400 milligrams. To give you some perspective, just one teaspoon of salt equals 2,300 milligrams of sodium.

The problem is, you may be consuming way too much sodium without even realizing it. "Americans eat a lot of sodium, much of it from convenience foods, bread products, and restaurant food, not just from the saltshaker on the table," warns Lindsey Pine, a registered dietitian nutritionist. Unfortunately, if you don't keep track of your daily sodium intake, you could unknowingly sabotage your heart health goals. A 2011 Northern Manhattan Study found that those who consume 4,000 mg per day, are two and a half times more likely to have a stroke than those who consumed less than 1,500 mg. "Those at risk for heart attack or stroke can benefit from a lower amount, usually between 1,500 mg-2000 mg, depending on the person and their lifestyle," recommends Pine.

Just as eliminating all unhealthy fats from your diet is nigh on impossible, the same holds true for sodium. Instead, look for ways to eliminate added sodium from the foods you eat:

- While scanning nutrition labels for unhealthy fats, keep an eye on the amount of sodium per serving.
- Flavor your own cooking with onions, garlic, vinegar, and spices. Just throw the table salt over your shoulder for good luck.
- When sitting down for dinner at a restaurant or friend's house, taste it first before reaching for the saltshaker. Not only can it be an insult to the cook if you salt it before taking a single bite, you may not need to salt it anyway.

Don't Forget to Sweat Your Stuff

The American Heart Association reports that lack of physical activity increases your risk of blood clots, high blood pressure, heart attack, and stroke. Adding physical activity is one of the most important improvements you can make on your journey to better heart health. The CDC, World Health Organization,

American Heart Association, and even yours truly agree that every adult aged 18-64 should try to get at least 150 minutes of moderate-intensity aerobic physical activity each week and strengthen your major muscle groups on two or more days per week.

How active are you in your daily life? If you like walking your dog, love ballroom dancing, enjoy housework (what is wrong with you?!), or head to the grocery store a couple of times a week, believe it or not, you are already participating in what the CDC labels as moderate activity. So, you might be shocked to know that when the CDC looked at data from the Behavioral Risk Factor Surveillance System in 2020, it found that, depending on where you live, 17.3 percent to 47.7 percent of adults in the United States report being physically inactive. No activity whatsoever? Who buys their groceries?

The good news is, your cardiovascular health doesn't discriminate the type of physical activity you choose, where you do it, and at what frequency. In Part Three of *Optimize Your Heart,* you'll learn how to start the exercise you enjoy, strategies for making it a habit, tips for breaking through stubborn fitness plateaus, and how to handle setbacks in your training. But, and this is the "but" that you may find the toughest when it comes to beginning any new exercise plan, you've got to get off your butt and get going.

Ready? Let's do this!

Application

Which of the above bad habits are you most guilty of? Start with small changes that will help you eventually eliminate them.

Part Three: Exercise Your Cardiac Muscle

10

Commencing to Begin

When you think of exercising you would be forgiven for immediately focusing on how it can help you lose weight and build muscle. After all, that's the message you constantly see on newsstands and in social media. While the external esthetics are one of the benefits earned from regular physical exercise, what happens on the inside is much more important.

As you exercise, your body delivers oxygen and nutrients to your muscles, brain, and tissues via your cardiovascular system. The more you exercise, the more efficient your heart becomes at circulating oxygen-rich blood, and over time both your blood pressure and resting heart rate are lowered. I could go deeper into the science of exercise and explain your aerobic, anaerobic, and phosphagen system, but you might decide it's time for a nap instead. Suffice to say your entire body benefits from regular exercise, but it's especially important for your cardiovascular health.

Just the Facts

Study after study shows that regular physical activity lowers your blood pressure, improves your cholesterol, helps you sleep, speeds up weight loss, and, ultimately, results in a reduced risk for a heart attack or stroke. A 2013 meta-analysis of 21 different studies found that increased levels of physical activity reduced the risk of heart disease by 21 percent in men and 29 percent in women.

The good news is, no matter your age, you will see a reduction in risk once you start adding regular exercise to your daily life. A 2011 study published in the Journal of the American College of Cardiology found that men who achieved high levels of fitness at age 45—and continued until their 80s—were four times less likely to die of heart disease over the course of their lifetime than those with low levels of fitness. Additionally, a study published in the European Heart Journal in 2019 showed that even if you wait until the age of 60, increasing activity levels can reduce your risk of cardiovascular disease by up to 11 percent!

So, what's stopping you from getting started with a new exercise regime, today, right this very minute? Sometimes that first step can be hard. So, let's set aside any fear of having to take one giant leap for mankind and instead start with a few baby steps.

Speak to Your Doctor, Again

If you've not already sat down with your primary care physician to discuss your heart health goals, now "might" be the time to make that appointment. I say "might" only because you may already have eye-rolled or hyperventilated at the thought of having to go back and see your doctor one more time. Until such time as your doctor tells you that you keep pestering them, you really can't call or meet with them too often. However, there is a simple form you can fill out to give you a better understanding of how necessary another appointment might be. It's called the PAR-Q.

The PAR-Q, a thankful abbreviation of the wordy Physical Activity Readiness Questionnaire, is a one-pager that uses seven questions to guide you as to whether you should speak to your doctor before you become more physically active. You can download a copy at www.AndyBeal.Fitness/optimize, but I'll give you a sneak peek at the questions:

1. Has your doctor ever said that you have a heart condition and that you should only do physical activity recommended by a doctor?
2. Do you feel pain in your chest when you do physical activity?

3. In the past month, have you had chest pain when you were not doing physical activity?
4. Do you lose your balance because of dizziness or do you ever lose consciousness?
5. Do you have a bone or joint problem (for example, back, knee, or hip) that could be made worse by a change in your physical activity?
6. Is your doctor currently prescribing drugs (for example, water pills) for your blood pressure or heart condition?
7. Do you know of any other reason why you should not do physical activity?

If you answer yes to any of these questions, then speak to your physician. Don't just take my word for it. Dr. Tina Harris, an internal medicine specialist, agrees. "I would recommend that patients speak to their doctor prior to starting an exercise regimen to determine their baseline level of fitness and design an exercise plan that accomplishes their goal whether it be weight loss, toning or cardiovascular fitness."

Don't be tempted to avoid that chat because you're worried your doctor may prevent you from exercising. I've had a heart attack and a stroke and even my cardiologist gave me the green light to train for a full marathon, 26.2 miles, because he knows my heart health like the back of his hand and is aware of all of my strengths and physical limitations. Which is impressive, as not everyone knows their own limitations, let alone someone else's.

Embrace Your Limitations

There may well be some exercise limitations that you simply cannot overcome. If you have already suffered a heart attack or stroke—my heart aches for you. Truly!—your doctor may rule out any kind of exercise other than instrumental activities of daily living, such as cleaning, bathing, laundry, or suggest a medically supervised program. "For patients with a recent heart attack, heart surgery, or a stroke, it would be recommended to begin an exercise regimen in a monitored setting such as cardiac rehabilitation," cautions Dr. Harris.

More likely, you have other physical, social, and environmental limitations that either make it hard for you to exercise or you've used as a mental crutch to justify your procrastination in using physical activity to improve your heart health. You can find ways to work around them.

If you have asthma, running may not be something you wish to consider, but you can still optimize your heart by walking or playing tennis. If you have a family, a home, two dogs, and a cat to take care of, a 60-minute kickboxing class might be hard to fit into your schedule, but 20-minutes on that elliptical machine—the one you previously reserved for drying clothes—is perfect! Whatever your limitations, accept them, embrace them, and adapt to them!

Get Going!

In the next chapter, you'll read guidance on the types of physical activity you can start in order to improve your heart health while having a relative modicum of fun. What you won't see are specific training plans for you to follow because, well, you are wonderfully unique, and you might hate me if I outlined a training plan for a 5K running race or suggested you do 30 burpees each day. (Okay, there's a minuscule chance you just tingled with excitement at the thought of doing burpees, but I am not willing to take that risk.)

Ready? Set? Go!

Application

Fill out the PAR-Q form. Nuff said.

11

Which Exercise is Best for You?

Like me, you've probably seen many articles and books that claim to have the magic answer to just about any question you have in life. If you're reading *Optimize Your Heart* looking for that one mythical exercise for improving your heart health, then let's go with burpees and call it a day. Not only am I kidding—burpees are miserable—but as a certified personal trainer, it would be very reckless of me to make assumptions about your goals, your limitations, or even your schedule. Instead, I am going to help you come up with your own magical exercise that will turn your inner spark of heart health improvement into a roaring fire of awesomeness!

To get you to that level, you'll first walk through six simple questions you can ask yourself while learning some practical advice along the way.

1. Aerobic, Strength, or Flexibility Training?

Do you already have a certain type of physical activity in mind? Nice! Is it aerobic in nature? Focused on strength training? Or, perhaps something designed to make you more flexible? In case you need a refresher, here's a quick summary of each:

Aerobic training – More commonly known as cardio, aerobic exercise is the type that primarily uses oxygen to turn carbs, proteins, and fats into energy. Typically performed at a light-to-moderate intensity, cardio includes physical activities such as swimming, jogging, elliptical training, cycling, tennis, and of course, any type of aerobics group class.

Strength training – When you think of strength training, you may immediately picture a gym with various weight machines, plates, and cables. That is indeed a major part of strength training, but it also includes bodyweight exercises such as pushups, squats, and planks. What they have in common is their focus on some kind of resistance force used to strengthen your muscles, bones, tendons, and joints.

Strength training is also where you can include some anaerobic exercise to build endurance. Anaerobic exercise favors glucose as a fuel over oxygen—anaerobic means without oxygen—and is more often found in high-intensity interval training, sprinting, and CrossFit.

Flexibility training – Flexibility training helps you to stretch muscles, improve your balance, and increase your freedom of movement. While you will find both cardio and strength training include some degree of stretching and balance, both tend to come up short as far as improving your suppleness and flexibility. That's where yoga, tai chi, and Pilates play an important role.

Okay, the quick overview is out of the way, but which type of exercise helps lower your risk for a heart attack or stroke? The answer is—drumroll please—all of them!

A 2002 study published in the British Medical Journal found that men who ran (cardio) for one hour or more each week reduced their risk for cardiovascular disease by 42 percent, while those who lifted weights (strength) for 30 minutes or more each week reduced their risk by 23 percent. And a paper published in the 2014 Indian Heart Journal demonstrated that yoga (flexibility) can reduce the risk of dying from a stroke by eight percent.

In an ideal world, you would try to include a little of each in your physical activities, but even an eight percent reduction in risk is a fantastic addition to your heart optimization plans.

2. What Matches Your Individual Needs?

You might have physical limitations that restrict the type of exercise options available to you. If you have osteoporosis, you'll prefer a physical activity that includes a lot of bodyweight strength training so you can build stronger bones. If you have a spinal cord injury, then you may hope to find a YMCA that offers wheelchair basketball.

You could simply have personal preferences. You dislike one-on-one personal training and instead thrive when surrounded by others in a group exercise class such as kickboxing or Zumba. The good news is, you can be very selective when it comes to finding the right physical activity for you. If having a baby goat on your back while doing a downward dog is your kind of exercise, then you'll likely find someplace, nearby, that is waiting for you to get started! I "kid" you not!

3. What Best Helps You Achieve Your Goal?

What's your current goal? No, I am not talking about your long-term motivation, as that should be to optimize your heart to reduce your risk for a stroke or heart attack. What I mean to ask is, what is your current SMART goal? The one you set back in Chapter 4?

If you want to enter a 5K race, then running is going to be an obvious choice, but even walking is a great place to start. Whereas lifting weights or attending a yoga class is not going to help you crush that goal in any meaningful way. If your goal is to be able to have the strength and flexibility to play outside with your grandchildren, then Pilates might be a better exercise than swimming.

The type of physical activity you choose should be the one that best helps you achieve that SMART goal.

4. Where Can You Exercise?

How close are you to a YMCA? Are there any bike trails near where you live? Do you have a rowing machine in your bonus room? This is just me trying to be clever, but really, I'm asking: where can you exercise?

If you have a gym in your apartment building, workplace, or your basement, then you might be all set when it comes to a location for your workouts. If not, then you had better jump on Yelp or ask your support network for recommendations for a great place to exercise. The key is to try and match your physical activity with something as close and convenient as possible. I would love to play badminton—I loved it in school—but the nearest location is 15 miles away, so I took up tennis instead. Your proximity to your physical activity of choice will greatly increase your adherence and turn something new into something you relish.

5. What Fits Your Schedule?

It can be hard to find a new physical activity that matches your interests, helps you achieve your goals, is close by, and also works with your schedule. When I studied martial arts, my school of choice had one huge deciding factor in its favor. Peck's Taekwondo offered lunchtime classes. At the stage, that was about the only time of day I could fit any exercise into my schedule. I had previously tried evening martial arts classes, but it was hard to fit into my schedule and so my dedication fizzled out after just four months. After joining Peck's Taekwondo, I studied for years and earned a second-degree black belt, primarily because I became a proud member of the Lunch Bunch group that trained and encouraged each other during midday classes.

In Chapter 12, you'll look at some ideas to help you schedule your workouts, but at this stage, you should keep in mind any scheduling conflicts or limitations which restrict your choice of physical activity. If you know there's no way you can fit in three trips to the local YMCA each week, but have space for a treadmill in your bedroom, then use that as means to achieve your half-marathon goal.

6. What Sounds the Most Fun?

Do you already feel a tingle of excitement and anticipation now that you have answered the above five questions? Hopefully, yes, but even if you feel your inner spark starting to fizzle out, I have one more question for you. And, I have saved the best for last:

What form of physical activity sounds the most fun to you?

If you only asked yourself one of the six questions, this should be the one. If you don't enjoy the exercise you use to improve your heart health, then likely you won't stick with it. You'll give it your best shot—like I did and failed with Pilates—but that desire to optimize your heart will only take you so far. When you pick a physical activity that sounds fun and you look forward to your next workout session, you not only improve your heart health, but also relieve stress, improve your mood, boost your confidence, increase your brain function, and even enhance your memory!

That doesn't mean you'll start like Olympian runner Usain Bolt out of the blocks. You still need to ease yourself into your new routine, track your progress, plan for any setbacks, and make sure you continue to fan your flame, even when life happens.

And it will happen. But, remember, life is what you're doing all of this for!

Application

Work through the six questions and make a short list of the physical activities that are most appealing. Try one, two, or even three and see which ones work best for you.

12

Your Health, Your Plan

If you Googled "150 minutes of exercise" you would see over 240 million results in the search engine's web index. The American Heart Association, the Centers for Disease Control and Prevention, the World Health Organization, even Britain's National Health Service are all on the same page when it comes to the amount of physical activity you should undertake each week:

> At least 150 minutes (2 hours and 30 minutes) of moderate-intensity aerobic activity (e.g. brisk walking, dancing, gardening) or 75 minutes (1 hour and 15 minutes) of vigorous-intensity activity (e.g. running, cycling, Zumba) each week (or an equivalent combination). Optionally, add at least two days a week of moderate to high-intensity strength training.

That can be easier read than done. Real life often gets in the way. Your schedule can get busy. Your motivation can dip. You may even feel overwhelmed at the mere thought of trying to add 150 minutes of exercise to a weekly routine that, up until 12 chapters ago, was comfortable and sedentary.

The good news is that any increase in physical activity is good for your heart health. In a 2015 Roundtable on Obesity Solutions discussion, experts suggested that simply adding 20 minutes of brisk walking each day can reduce the risk of death by 24 percent in people of normal weight and by 16 percent in people who are obese. And you can further divide that up into two 10-minute walks each day and achieve the same reduction in risks.

Now all you need to do is find a way to build up to 150 minutes or more of moderate physical activity each week.

Start Quickly, Build Slowly

Just like I wouldn't recommend you overhaul your diet in just one week—remember, make small, healthy food switches first—I would not recommend anyone who has previously been inactive suddenly push for 150 minutes of moderate exercise in their first week. Instead, start slowly—both the length of time for each exercise and the intensity. Jim Burrows, an avid runner and high school cross country and track coach, tells aspiring runners to start with walking. "Your body needs time to adapt to your new hobby. Walking gets the body used to moving and after a week or two you'll be ready to transition to run/walks."

The best rule of thumb is to increase your physical activity by five to ten percent each week. This is something that personal trainers call progression. Progression applies to the duration of your physical activity (10 minutes to 11 minutes), the distance (1 mile to 1.1 miles), difficulty (10-pound weight to 11-pound weight), etc., etc. Not only will small increases make it more practical for fitting exercise into your weekly schedule, but they will also help you avoid fatigue and injuries caused by over-training and pushing your body too hard, too fast.

Schedule Your Successes

Now that you have a good idea of the amount of physical activity that makes the most sense to your body, it's time to flex that index finger and tap, swipe, or turn the page in your calendar.

What time of day? – Are you a morning, afternoon, or evening person? If you find yourself with unlimited energy at 6 a.m. each morning—kudos for getting your seven hours of sleep—then your weight training will be much more productive at that time compared to tacking it on after a long day of work. Choose the time of day that best matches your highest energy levels.

What days of the week? – If you only have two mornings a week free for exercise, you'll be far more energized and committed to your new physical activity if you schedule those two mornings than if you reluctantly tried to squeeze in workouts at night. Pick the days of the week that have the best availability for your preferred time of day.

What matches mutual availability? – If you plan to walk on the treadmill in your spare room, then you are blessed with a situation that allows you to schedule your physical activity solely around your availability. If you want to join a group yoga class or hire a personal trainer, then you'll need to find a mutually convenient time. If looking for a class, meetup, or personal trainer, shop around. I have two YMCA locations near me, and each has the same type of classes but at different times and on different days.

Schedule it! – How many times have you missed a doctor's appointment? Or failed to show up at your annual performance review? I would guess less than one percent of the time because, when you have something important coming in the week ahead, you make a note of the time and place in your calendar. Your heart health is just as important, and so you should add your workouts to your calendar. You will be less likely to forget or avoid a workout because you accidentally-on-purpose scheduled coffee with a friend at the same time.

Professionals Provide Personalized Plans

With your new workout timeslots planned in your calendar, it's time to figure out the best structure for that allotted time. This is often where a personal trainer, physical therapist, or sports coach bring a host of benefits.

Planning your development – When I first started strength training, I hired my own personal trainer, Perry Junior. A U.S. Navy veteran, he's a certified personal trainer, and physique bodybuilder. If anyone could get my heart in shape it was him! I was a newbie to strength training and had little idea what I needed to do to lose weight and gain muscle. Fortunately, Junior started me on a training plan that focused on a mix of aerobic, flexibility, and strength training.

Mixing things up – Some personal trainers will tell you that you should mix up your strength training to keep your muscles surprised and guessing. That's a bit of a stretch of what science has proven. What *is* true is that when you hire someone to design and oversee your workouts, they will keep each session fun and challenging. Junior explains, "I never give my clients the same workout, so they arrive at each session with a sense of excitement and anticipation."

Keeping you accountable – Even if you don't feel like you need a coach or trainer watching your every move, having someone to hold you accountable will increase your adherence to your new exercise schedule.

After I set up a weekly exercise plan for a client, I check in with them after each workout to see how it went, encourage them, guide them, but also keep them accountable. It may sound harsh, but the feedback I get is that they appreciate knowing if they skip a workout, they will have to 'fess up. Which means they rarely miss a scheduled workout.

Doing the heavy lifting – Another good reason to hire a personal trainer or sports coach is that they do a lot of the heavy lifting for you. No, I don't mean they are the ones who lift the barbell on your behalf, although they will help if needed. You pay them, so they are the ones who make sure everything is set up, sanitized, and efficient. I've taken many tennis lessons at the Raleigh Racquet Club and never have to worry about booking a court, bringing balls, or making sure the clay is cleaned and groomed for play.

Adherence Deserves a Reward

When you set up your SMART goal you likely focused on the outcome you most desired. Lose 20 pounds, improve your blood pressure, or run a 5K, but you can additionally set goals that are aligned with your calendar. If you've scheduled your week to include walking for 20 minutes each day and two 25-minute strength training sessions, then why not make adhering to that plan an additional goal?

Motivate yourself with the promise of a new pair of walking shoes, a nice massage, or some other prize that further encourages you to keep exercising. Remember, when you set your own reward for achieving any goal, you are 50 percent more likely to achieve that goal than if you didn't have that enticing, nutritious carrot dangling in front of you.

Let Me Get Back to You on That

What if you have to miss a workout because your boss called you in early for a team meeting? Or you have a goal of losing 30 pounds before the end of the year, but discover that Thanksgiving and Christmas are once again going to be celebrated in November and December? So rude! A common response is to throw your hands up in the air and decide that you should just scrap your exercise plans because the universe is conspiring against you. Well, I am sorry to give you a wake-up call, but life happens.

There have been many times when my pre-scheduled workout was interrupted by some unforeseen event that meant I could not complete it. My two normal responses are to either shrug it off and just get right back on schedule for my next planned workout, or I improvise something. Living room push-ups, a quick neighborhood walk, or grab the kettlebell and swing it between client calls. What I have never done is to use it as a metaphorical note from my mom that I can no longer continue with my plans to improve my heart health.

You will always face setbacks, unexpected events, and failures. The key is how you respond. As the late Jim Valvano, former North Carolina State University basketball coach, is famous for saying, "Don't give up, don't ever give up!"

Keep moving forward.

Application

If you need help setting up your exercise schedule, head to www.AndyBeal.Fitness/optimize to download a free training plan.

13

Do Sweat the Small Stuff

"Get six-pack abs fast!", "Run a faster 5K!", "Take this supplement for massive muscle growth!" If you scan the magazine covers of Men's Health, Shape, or Muscle & Fitness, you will very likely see similar headlines. Over and over again. The reason being they want you to read and so they focus on the topics that have the broadest appeal. Who doesn't want six-pack abs?

I'm only being passively-aggressively critical of the abundance of this type of information when it comes to physical fitness. It certainly has its place. However, there are dozens of small, valuable exercise tips that I wish I had discovered sooner. I can't unpack every one of the lesser-shared tips I have learned over the years in just one chapter, but I can share the ones which I believe will help you to succeed in your new plan to optimize your heart.

Record Your Benchmarks

Whenever you set out to improve your health, you need to record your starting point against which you will measure your progress. If you want to become an elite bodybuilder, measuring your body fat percentage and the size of your biceps would be high on your list of benchmark measurements. More realistically, your main desire is to reduce your risk of cardiovascular disease while also reaching your SMART goal, so you should consider taking the following measurements:

- Your resting heart rate.
- Your resting blood pressure.
- Your blood sugar.
- Your waist size.
- Your weight.

Of course, you can add any other measurements that are important to you, but those are the primary ones that, when improved, will give you a warm and fuzzy feeling about your heart health.

Also, take some photos of yourself. Did you just cringe? I know I did when I took some photos of myself at my heaviest weight ever. I couldn't even bring myself to smile. You don't need to post them to Instagram, but if you take them and save them to your phone, or 256-bit encrypted hard drive that no one can access but you, you will be thrilled you did at some point.

Nothing makes you feel quite as amazing as comparing your new, optimized self against your old photos. And you will likely want to share that comparison online. Yes, it gives your ego a small massage but, more importantly, your before and after photos might inspire someone else to improve their physical fitness.

Assess Yourself So You Don't Wreck Yourself

Your next step is to do some kind of physical assessment. There are dozens of different types of fitness assessments that you could use and ideally you would work with a personal trainer, physical therapist, or if you have previously suffered a stroke or heart attack, a cardiac rehab team. If they are not part of your physical activity plans, then consider the following self-assessments:

- **Aerobic fitness:** How long does it take you to walk one mile?
- **Upper body strength:** How many push-ups can you do to failure?
- **Lower body strength:** How many squats can you do to failure?
- **Flexibility:** Seated on the floor, legs fully extended in front, how far forward can you reach with your fingers?

You should adapt your fitness assessment to suit your physical limitations, chosen physical activity, and SMART goal. For example, if you plan to swim laps at your local pool, then consider switching out the one-mile walk test with the number of yards you can currently swim.

By conducting an initial self-assessment, you will be able to create a training plan that improves upon your existing level of fitness. Conduct the same assessments each month so you can see your improvements and maybe make any reward conditional upon making progress.

Gear Up!

There's something about investing in new exercise gear that psychologically fires you up for your next workout. Some brand-new running shoes, a moisture-wicking shirt, or a brightly colored exercise mat. The options are endless. Here's what to look for:

- Buy what best matches your chosen physical activity. Running shoes serve a different purpose than hiking shoes.
- Be frugal with your initial purchase. When I first started Pilates, I bought a mat and that was it. I used the YMCA's exercise balls and Pilates rings until I could be sure that I would enjoy the classes and stick with it.
- Shop sales or buy gently used equipment. Look for last year's clearance model or browse your local Play It Again Sports store.

At the end of the day, treat yourself to whatever fits your budget and helps you look forward to your next workout. Just don't be tempted to buy an entirely new wardrobe, a carbon-fiber triathlon bike, or the same model tennis racquet used by Roger Federer, until you know you love your new physical activity, it fits your schedule, and you have turned it into a regular habit. In other words, wait 66 days!

Fuel Up!

Psst! Want to know the one thing you should consume to get the most out of your physical activity? According to actor Adam Sandler, it's some "high-quality H2O." If you've never watched the movie "Waterboy," my joke will be lost on you, but the answer is still accurate. Drink water!

Make sure you bring water along with you for any physical activity that lasts longer than 20 minutes. When you exercise, you sweat. If the air temperature is hot, you will sweat some more. If you don't replace your lost fluids, you will get dehydrated, which can lead to muscle cramps, fatigue, dizziness, and in extreme cases, heatstroke.

As you progress from moderate physical activity to something more vigorous, you can learn more about the benefits of carb-loading, protein shakes, electrolytes, and energy gels. For now, stay hydrated and consider watching "Waterboy" after your next workout. You can do it!

Streeetch!

Flexibility training involves a mix of stretching, mobility, and balancing. Even if your new workout schedule focuses mostly on aerobic or strength training, stretching before and after is vitally important.

Before your workout, warm up with some dynamic stretches. Dynamic stretching is designed to warm up your muscles and tissue in preparation for your physical activity. Walking lunges, arm circles, and high kicks are all examples of dynamic stretching. In a nutshell, lightly move your body to warm up your muscles and reduce the risk of injury.

After you have exercised, cool down with some static stretches. Static stretches are designed to help loosen up muscles that naturally become tight and sore after any physical activity. Grabbing your ankle and pulling your foot up to your buttock, pulling one arm across your body, and sitting on the floor, feet straight out, and reaching for your toes, are all examples of static stretching.

You may be tempted to skip both dynamic and static stretching. You would not be alone. However, there's a good reason why you should include stretching in your warm-up and cool-down. A 2020 study published in The Journal of Physiology followed men and women over a 12-week stretching program and found that those who engaged in stretching had increased blood flow and decreased arterial stiffness. That's a pretty compelling heart-healthy reason!

Start Slow for Fast Results

Have you ever seen a beginner swinging really heavy weights in the gym? It looks impressive, but then they either tire quickly or worse, injure themselves. You may see something similar with new runners. They sprint out of their imaginary starting blocks, but once they turn the corner and you can no longer see them, they run out of gas and grab the back of their cramping calf muscle. A lot of times, those new to any physical activity simply try to do too much at the beginning.

By starting cardio slowly or lifting lighter weights, there are many benefits, including:

- You will quickly gauge your current capability and then increase the intensity as needed.
- Warm up your muscles to your new workout and reduce the chance of injury.
- You can focus on your technique and whether you are performing the exercise correctly.

No matter your chosen type of physical exercise—aerobic, strength, or flexibility—start slowly so that you can listen to how your body is responding.

Listen to Your Body

One of the best ways to measure whether your exercise intensity matches your current fitness level is by using the Rate of Perceived Exertion, or RPE, scale. RPE is designed to measure the intensity of your workout on a scale of one to ten. During any physical activity, ask yourself your current RPE. If you answer 1, then you probably just made a trip to the bathroom and back. Not exactly a meaningful physical activity. If you answer with a 10, you were probably just chased by a mountain lion. If you're hoping to perform some type of moderate physical activity, then your rate of perceived exertion should feel like a 5 or a 6, while vigorous activity should be closer to a 7 or 8.

Self-monitoring with the RPE scale can also act as an early warning sign that you might be pushing your body too far. If you ever feel like you're scoring a 9 or 10, you should scale back. Check your pulse and, if you have a cuff, your blood pressure. It is normal for exercise to elevate both, but an extremely elevated pulse or blood pressure is one of the many signs that you should stop your current workout and speak to your doctor.

Know When to Stop

I am in the best shape of my life. I have run half-marathons, played three-hour tennis matches, and today I rode my mountain bike for over an hour, and then completed a full-body strength training workout. And yet, I am constantly watching for any warning signs that I should stop my workout immediately. These are the ones you should watch for:

- Feeling a squeezing, burning, or tightness under your breastbone that spreads to your left arm or shoulder, back, or jaw. These are common signs of angina (reduced blood flow to your heart).
- Feeling lightheaded, confused, or dizzy.
- Unusual or extreme shortness of breath.
- Your heartbeat feels fast, uneven, or skips.
- Severe cramping or numbness in any of your muscles.

If you experience any of the above or indeed feel anything out of the ordinary, don't prioritize a new personal record over and above your health. Stop exercising immediately. If you start feeling better right away, then schedule a future visit with your physician just to be safe. If the symptoms persist, even after you've stopped exercising, take a trip to the emergency room.

Remember, your goal is to optimize your heart. When it comes to exercise, this means making smart adjustments that allow you to improve your cardiovascular system. Along the way, plateaus will happen, goals might be missed, but any improvement to your heart health is something to celebrate.

Application

Make a note of your benchmarks and while conducting your first assessment, stay in an RPE range of 5 to 6.

14

Reach the Peak of Your Success

Congratulations! After weeks of improving your physical health, it's now time for you to celebrate reaching your fitness...plateau!

"Wait, what? How is that something to celebrate?" you might be asking. When you experience plateaus in your physical fitness, you might focus on the fact that your weight loss has stopped, you can't run much faster, or your resting blood pressure just isn't improving any further. All potentially demoralizing. Yet, if you revisit what plateau really means, you might be greatly encouraged. Oxford Languages' definition of plateau is "Reach a state of little or no change after a time of activity or progress."

The plateau effect is something worth celebrating. You have engaged in a new physical activity, exercise class, or sport and have worked hard to make progress.

You have now reached your personalized peak of success!

Success Served on a Plateau

Remember, *Optimize Your Heart* is about helping you make small changes to reduce your risk for a heart attack or stroke. If you were in perfect physical health, able to transform into an elite athlete, you probably wouldn't even be reading this book. Instead, accept there are many reasons why you may have hit your peak earlier than you expected.

Your family history – Your inherited risk factors or physical limitations might limit the peak level of physical fitness you can achieve. With my asthma, I can run 13.2 miles, but at a pace that some elite runners would consider a brisk walk.

Your body wants your attention – If you reach a plateau that doesn't make sense to you, then your doctor can help answer your body's riddle. Perhaps your cortisol levels are too high, your thyroid is underactive, or one of your medications is causing your unexplained weight gain, fatigue, or muscle pain.

Your body's not ready – A plateau doesn't have to be permanent, but to break through it, you may have to increase your intensity, frequency, or weight. Be patient. It could take you weeks, months, or even years before you're ready to move on to your next peak.

You're perfectly happy – There's a fine line between exercise for fitness and exercise for performance. If a Pilates class twice a week is enough to keep you happy, motivated, and committed to exercise, that is much better than pushing yourself so hard that you burn out after just four weeks and return to the couch.

Compare Yourself to Your Old Self

Now that you feel better about reaching your peak, it's a good time to remind yourself of just how much you have improved your physical fitness. Some of the best ways to do that include:

Take your measurements again – Whichever benchmark measurements you took at the outset, take again. Maybe they haven't all improved, but even just a quarter-inch off your waist or two pounds of lost weight have you heading in the right direction towards reducing your risk for a heart attack or stroke.

Take a new photo – Sometimes improvements happen so slowly, and so subtly, they go unnoticed. Taking a new photo might reveal that your skin looks smoother and less wrinkled because you are drinking more water and sleeping better than ever before.

Reassess your physical fitness – Perhaps you'll discover you can walk at a faster rate than when you started. You can now physically touch your toes, instead of just waving to them. And, any increase in the number of push-ups you can do is awesome! If you do thrive on extreme goals, a study in the 2019 JAMA Network Open found that men able to do 40 push-ups or more lowered their risk for cardiovascular disease by 96 percent!

It can be tempting to look around a sports club or gym and compare your level of physical fitness to those around you, but remember, measure your optimized self against your old self, not others.

There is a Magical Exercise, After All

If you've spoken to your doctor, improved your diet, quit smoking, or increased the amount of sleep you get each night, you have already taken a valuable step towards optimizing your heart. Increasing the amount of physical activity in your life is just one of the many improvements you can make to your heart health. If, after everything you have read in Part Three of *Optimize Your Heart*, you are still struggling to find the time and motivation to increase your physical activity, please consider trying this one last strategy: go for a walk.

My mother-in-law has a long family history of heart disease. Her father died of cardiac arrest. Her mother had a stroke. And, three of her brothers experienced heart attacks. Those were enough warning signs for her to realize she needed to optimize her heart health.

Not having the interest to join a gym or keep up to date with the latest exercise trends, she resolved to walk more. She walked around her yard, driveway, even up and down her home's hallway, to reduce her risk of a heart attack or stroke. Now, in her seventies, walking daily continues to keep her blood pressure in check, her total cholesterol low, and impresses her doctor enough that she doesn't need a cardiac stress test each year.

Success is Just Ten Minutes Away

It seems fitting that I end with one last positive research study. Published in the 2017 Journal of the American College of Cardiology, researchers looked at 15,486 patients with heart disease and found that those who went for a 10-minute brisk walk each day had a 33 percent lower risk of death than those who had no physical activity.

You can start with ten minutes of walking a day. I believe in you!

Application

You guessed it, put down Optimize Your Heart and go for a 10-minute brisk walk.

Conclusion

If, like me, you are the type of book reader who always skips ahead to the Conclusion to get a sneak-peek of how the author sums up their advice, then I am sorry to say you will be disappointed. This Conclusion can't reveal what YOU need to do to improve your health and prevent a heart attack or stroke. The reason being, all 14 chapters of *Optimize Your Heart* are designed to help you personally navigate the many different ways you can reduce your risk of, or even reverse, cardiovascular disease. Only you know which changes will work best for your heart.

There's a plethora of science that I could have shared with you, but you likely would have found it dry, overwhelming, and well, preachy. Having your daily diet for the next four weeks spelled out in detail is common in many books, but also inspired by the author's tastes and not yours. I don't know about you, but every time I see cantaloupe, cucumber, or olives listed, I immediately stop reading and go sob in a corner. Likewise, giving you the precise blood pressure or HDL cholesterol number you should achieve wouldn't factor in your genetics, physical limitations, and challenges of daily life.

Instead, my goal, my desire, is to provide you with some proven advice, a helpful nudge, and point you in the right direction. I have faced what you may be facing—the dreaded thought that I am at risk of someday having a heart attack or stroke. I didn't dodge either of those bullets, but thankfully, I did start making small improvements early enough that when I stared down a stroke, heart attack, and coronary heart disease, each of which could have left me dead, I recovered. Not only did I recover, I thrived. I continue to make small changes. I continue to enjoy small indulgences. I don't measure myself against what the researchers and doctors tell me. I measure myself against my old self and realize that I have come a long way in my efforts to optimize my heart.

Now is the time for you to start your journey. Remember, don't feel pressured to rush into this. It took you decades to get to where you are today. Not only is an overnight change impossible, but attempting such a dramatic overhaul would mean taking the beautiful work of art your current life represents and whitewashing it clean. Don't do it. Instead, look for the changes you can make that are small enough that you can stick with them. Any improvement to your diet, exercise, medication, sleep, or stress level will help improve your cardiovascular health. Add another change. And another. Over time, you'll feel better, look better, and your heart will beat better.

I have just one favor to ask. When you are done absorbing all of the advice in this book, please leave a review on Amazon so that someone else—someone who is struggling with the looming reality that they, too, may one day experience a stroke or heart attack—might learn how *Optimize Your Heart* can improve their cardiovascular health.

May it encourage and guide them, as much as I hope it has you.

God bless.

Appendix A: Know the Signs

Stroke

A stroke occurs when a blood vessel to the brain either bursts or is blocked by a clot. When this occurs, part of the brain cannot receive the oxygen-rich blood it needs, and brain cells start to die.

Learn the FAST acronym to help identify a stroke:

Face Drooping – Does one side of the face droop or is it numb? Does a smile droop on one side of the mouth?
Arm Weakness – When both arms are raised, is one weak, drifting down, or completely numb?
Speech – Is speech slurred, unable to repeat a simple sentence or answer questions?
Time to Call 911 – If any of the above symptoms exist, get to the hospital as quickly as possible.

Heart Attack

A heart attack is when the blood flow to the heart is blocked. If the blocked artery is not reopened quickly, that part of the heart can die.

Learn the PULSE acronym to help identify a heart attack:

> **P**ain in the chest, neck, back, jaw, or arms
> **U**pset stomach, including nausea, indigestion, or vomiting
> **L**ightheadedness or dizziness
> **S**hortness of breath
> **E**xcessive sweating

What to do:

- Call 911 immediately.

Cardiac Arrest

Cardiac arrest is when the heart has an electrical malfunction and suddenly stops beating.

Warning signs:

- The heart has stopped beating and there is no pulse.
- A loss of consciousness.

What to do:

- Call 911 immediately.
- Perform hands-only CPR (Cardiopulmonary Resuscitation). Place hands on chest and push hard and fast to the beat of the disco song "Stayin' Alive" until the pulse returns or paramedics arrive.

Appendix B: Resources

American Heart Association – https://www.heart.org/

American Stroke Association – https://www.stroke.org/

Centers for Disease Control and Prevention – https://www.cdc.gov/heartdisease/index.htm

Office on Women's Health – https://www.womenshealth.gov/heart-disease-and-stroke/

World Heart Federation – https://www.world-heart-federation.org/

American College of Cardiology – https://www.cardiosmart.org/

Smokefree – https://smokefree.gov/

CPR and First Aid – https://cpr.heart.org/

Andy Beal, Cardiac Prehab Personal Trainer – https://andybeal.fitness/

~~Acknowledgments~~ Appreciation

Just like my last book, *Repped*, the inspiration for *Optimize Your Heart* was a gift from God. Fittingly, the idea, outline, and title for the book came to me while walking around my neighborhood. I never thought I would find a reason to write another book, but it found me.

My wife, Sheila, has always provided me with tremendous support while I have my head down researching and writing my books. This time, not only did she show patience and encouragement during the creation of *Optimize Your Heart*, but she enthusiastically took on the role of providing the initial copy edits and pointed out improvements in readability. If you found the book easy to follow, be sure to thank her when you see her! The final manuscript was once again sent over to the ever-helpful Lisa Lickel for her proofreading and style suggestions.

My sincere appreciation also goes out to all of the doctors, nurses, and caregivers at Duke Health, WakeMed, and UNC REX Healthcare. Not only are they instrumental in my improved cardiovascular health, but tirelessly help thousands of heart attack and stroke patients each year.

A very special thanks to Omar Kass-Hout M.D. who started as my newly assigned neurologist, but quickly jumped on board and offered to write the excellent foreword for this book.

Lastly, I would like to thank my family, friends, clients, and even strangers, who have prayed for me, supported me, and encouraged me.

My sincere thanks and appreciation to you all!

Index

About the Author

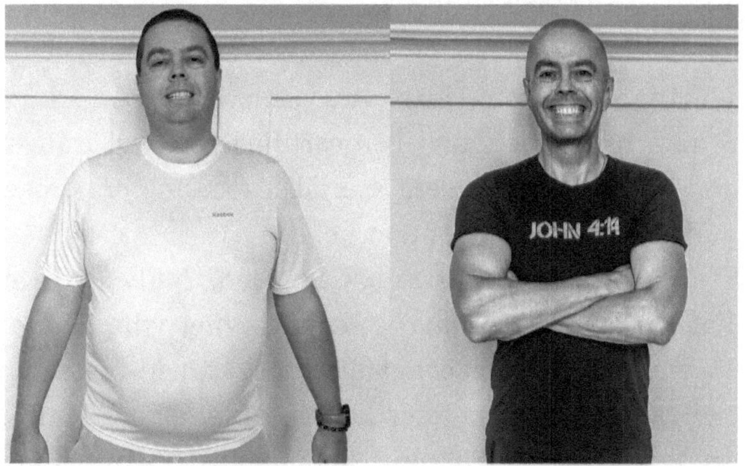

Andy Beal is known as both The Original Online Reputation Expert™ as well as the Cardiac Prehab Personal Trainer™. As the CEO of Reputation Refinery, Andy authored two books on the topic of online reputation management: *Repped* and *Radically Transparent*, and has helped individuals, companies, and audiences worldwide.

In 2018, at the age of 44, Andy suffered a massive stroke and a minor heart attack. The stroke could have paralyzed his entire right side. Thankfully, Andy made a decision eight months earlier to improve his cardiovascular health. His commitment to optimize his heart health contributed to what doctors call a "remarkable recovery" and his health transformation was featured by the American Heart Association, ABC11, and Men's Health.

Andy now spends his spare time as an ambassador for the American Heart Association, the American Stroke Association, and is a certified personal trainer and weight management specialist focusing on stroke and heart attack prevention.

Originally from Brighton, England, Andy lives in Raleigh, North Carolina with his loving wife, Sheila. When not helping companies build their brand or individuals optimize their health, Andy enjoys tennis, mountain biking, running, and fueling up by eating salmon salads. If you can't find Andy on the courts, trails, or social media, look for him giving thanks to God at Providence Baptist Church.

If you would like Andy to personally help you improve your heart health, please visit www.AndyBeal.Fitness.